Praise for Twins: a practical and emotional guide to parenting twins

This book covers just about every relevant subject from insurance to bereavement. If I had twins I'd buy it.

Lucy Sussex, *The Sunday Age*

I would like to congratulate you both on compiling such an excellent, informative and realistic account of the joys and difficulties of having twins.

Cathy Vellacott, Vice CEO AMBA

Far from being the horror story that most books make multiple pregnancies out to be, this book is honest and informative. It does not shy away from the risks, but addresses them as possible rather than inevitable.

Sue Mulrennan, NZMBA

I used some precious sleep time last night to read *Twins* and quite frankly could not put it down. I wish I had something like this to read when I was pregnant – it's so comprehensive, practical and easy to read. It is Australian, recent and down to earth – a warts-and-all look at parenting twins which is very refreshing and reassuring.

Michelle Moore, Bellingen NSW

I was told by AMBA about this book and found it to be a godsend! I have read it two times now … I am now 24 weeks pregnant with twins and being a first time mother there were things I had not thought about this early. I'm extremely grateful that we had the chance to discuss things now and not during labour where every second counts.

Tennille Telford

It was great hearing the turmoil that other twin parents have gone through too so I didn't feel like it was just happening to me, and that others have done it before me, and harder too. We were going through hard times with them when I bought the book and I was so tired, yet I just had to read it. It was inspirational.

Kylie Beatson

You should be proud of yourselves for writing an insightful and realistic book that can be of help to so many women. Especially to the ones out in the bush like me who are oblivious to the facts and figures regarding multiple births.

Stephanie Renton.

Thankyou, thankyou, thankyou for writing this book. It literally saved my boys' lives and made mine a little more bearable … If we hadn't have read your book or had waited until the obstetrician had returned from holiday in 6 days time, [my cholestasis would have gone undiagnosed and] we would have lost our babies. Unthinkable.

Yolande Dickinson-Smith, Wellington, New Zealand

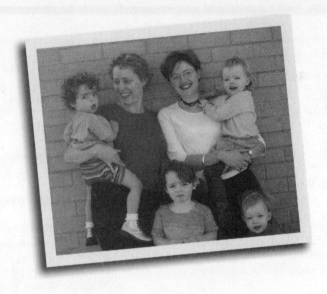

Katrina Bowman and Louise Ryan met at a
South Eastern Multiple Birth Association barbecue,
bonded instantly, and within weeks were writing the book
they wished they'd had when pregnant with their twins.

Katrina works part-time as a communications
consultant and her girls, Charlotte and Ella Hart,
were born in 2000. Louise works full-time in sales and marketing
and her girls, Celeste and Camille, were born in 1999.

TWINS

**A practical guide to parenting multiples
from conception to preschool**

Katrina Bowman and Louise Ryan

A Sue Hines Book

ALLEN & UNWIN

First published in Australia in 2002
This revised edition first published in Australia in 2005

A Sue Hines Book
Allen & Unwin
83 Alexander Street
Crows Nest NSW 2065
Australia
Phone: (61 2) 8425 0100
Fax: (61 2) 9906 2218
Email: info@allenandunwin.com
Web: www.allenandunwin.com

National Library of Australia
Cataloguing-in-Publication entry:

Bowman, Katrina, 1968– .
    Twins: a practical guide to parenting multiples from conception to preschool.

    Rev. ed.
    Bibliography.
    Includes index.
    ISBN 1 74114 653 4.

    1. Twins. 2. Multiple pregnancy. 3. Multiple birth. 4. Parenting. 5. Child rearing.
    I. Ryan, Louise, 1962– . II. Title.

    649.144

Cover & text design by Studio Pazzo
Cover illustration by Andrea McNamara
Typeset by Pauline Haas

Edited by Jenny Lord

Index by Fay Donlevy

Printed by Griffin Press, South Australia

10 9 8 7 6 5 4 3 2 1

Contents

Foreword

Since establishing Australia's first Multiple Pregnancy Clinic in 1997, I have been involved in the care of more than 500 couples expecting twins, triplets or quadruplets. My patients, both in the Multiple Pregnancy Clinic, and in my private Obstetric practice, have struggled to find adequate information resources for Australian women expecting a multiple birth. Thankfully, this is no longer the case.

Katrina and Louise have extensively researched the area of twin pregnancy and written with experience and good humour to produce the definitive guide to parenting twins.

Not only have they provided a much needed Australian flavour to the subject, but they have provided an invaluable resource to parents everywhere.

As well as providing a thoughtful and sensible guide to parenting twins, they have also confronted many difficult issues. The sections on coping with limited resources, foetal reduction and depression should prove particularly helpful for those faced with these situations.

The medical information is carefully and accurately presented and cleverly interspersed with parental experiences. The result is a book that is not only easy to read but is an excellent reference tool.

Twins: A practical guide to parenting multiples from conception to pre-school should be compulsory reading not only for women expecting twins but their partners, family and friends.

Dr Mark Umstad
Obstetrician and Gynaecologist
Head of Multiple Pregnancy Clinic,
The Royal Women's Hospital, Melbourne

Before you read on

Congratulations on achieving minor celebrity status as parents or potential parents of twins or triplets. You will be stopped in the streets more often than you can imagine and asked about your darling babies. This is some small acknowledgement of how lucky you are. You *are* lucky, but you're also going to be very busy!

When we found out that we were expecting twins, both of us wanted to find out everything we possibly could about what was happening to our bodies and babies so we could get ready, but we found that mainstream support systems concentrated on people having one baby at a time. It is very special to be parents of twins yet despite the increasing frequency of multiple births the written information available on multiple pregnancy, birth and parenting was scarce.

So we collected information from every source we could think of. Conversations with parents of multiples became interviews. We advertised in multiples' newsletters to find people with different experiences, surfed the Internet and rang organisations who deal with aspects of multiples issues. We read every available book on the subject. The result is a mix of medical, practical, emotional and anecdotal information, a great reference for tired, busy people.

The arrival of multiples places a huge strain on you and your relationships – you will experience physical, emotional and financial demands that are often greater than parenting one baby at a time. The stories we have included range from shocking to inspirational, from reassuring to heartbreaking – emotional turmoil is a significant part of parenting twins. Our own stories are honest accounts of our experiences because we wanted to share the good and the bad, including our 'mistakes'. You get the benefit of our hindsight.

At an AMBA national convention, a number of parents of triplets asked us to include their concerns in the next edition of *Twins*. Because we had no direct experience of having three babies at once, a big thank you to the triplet parents who shared their stories for *Twins: a practical guide to parenting multiples from conception to preschool*.

Being organised is crucial to parents of multiples and since you're reading this book, you're off to a good start, having information at your fingertips. So read on ...

We welcome feedback and we'd be delighted to hear of different experiences and any suggestions for our next edition of *Twins: a practical guide to parenting multiples from conception to preschool.*

twinsbook@bigpond.com

Thanks to all the families who emailed us with feedback for this revised edition.

There's a pair in there

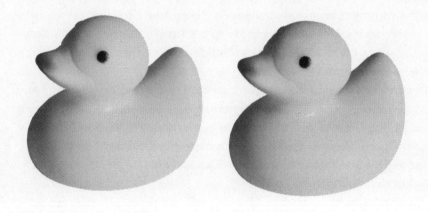

FINDING OUT IT'S TWINS

FINDING OUT IT'S TWINS: OUR STORIES

In the past many women didn't know they were having twins until the birth. We're now most likely to find out well before our babies are born. Doctors sometimes find twins when they're checking for a heartbeat and hear two, or by feeling two heads through your abdomen. Usually the discovery is made during an ultrasound at any time between six and 20 weeks. If you've had fertility treatment, earlier miscarriages, bleeding or any other reason to be concerned, you may be given an ultrasound scan at around six weeks (where two tiny heartbeats may be detected). Ultrasound scans for a naturally conceived twin pregnancy are usually done between 18 and 20 weeks.

You may have suspected you were having two babies before it was confirmed by ultrasound. Sometimes it's because of extreme sickness, especially when you can compare it to an earlier pregnancy or because you seem larger than expected or have put on a lot of weight. Or you may have had no idea.

Katrina: Are you sure you're not having twins, you're big for 20 weeks, was the comment from a wry colleague. There aren't any twins in my family; I just had a bit of padding there to start with, was my equally light-hearted reply. My sister and I joked the day before the ultrasound that if it's twins she can have one of them.

At our first ultrasound the technician kept remarking on how the baby was moving around a lot. I was very eager for confirmation that we were having a girl. Then he said it. There are two babies. We laughed; surely he was joking. He showed us the screen and pointed out two heads.

I spoke my first thought. 'Are they Siamese?'

'What do you mean by Siamese?'

'Stuck together.'

'There's nothing to indicate that.'

I burst into tears.

'It's not that I don't love them,' I tell my husband. 'I'm just a bit shocked. How will we ever cope with two?' He reassures me, 'We'll do it together.'

On the way home in the car the tears were still flowing and I realised I was wrong. I didn't love them. I didn't want them. I didn't want two babies. It was too late for a termination. Perhaps I'd lose them. How would we ever manage? How could I have been so unlucky?

I have always felt sorry for twins. Having someone who looks just like you, always competing with you. They lose their individuality. I didn't want my children to have that.

I had always wanted children. We delayed it for some years, then when I decided it was time we managed to conceive first try, much to my husband's disappointment! If I'd known I was going to have twins, I thought, I would have really questioned having children. Still, it had been my decision to have a baby. This was actually my fault. What had I done?

I had an instant and desperate need to know more about twins and how we could raise them as individuals. We spent the evening researching. It appeared from the scan that our twins were probably identical, which is not genetic, just a one in 250 chance. It was my egg that had split. Perhaps I shouldn't have jumped in that hot tub? Did heat cause eggs to split? This really is my fault. That seed of self-blame was planted.

I quickly realised that a large part of my distress was grief. I was grieving for the loss of a single baby. For years I held in my mind's eye a peaceful image of me rocking my baby in the sunshine. But now I was not going to have any peace, no one-on-one close contact. I felt I was being denied time to love my children. I would be too busy just coping. I felt very sorry for myself.

I knew I had no right to moan. It wasn't like someone had died. My babies appeared healthy. I shouldn't have felt like this. I should have been over the moon. What was wrong with me? Why was this happening?

Louise: Getting pregnant is an accident for some couples, easy for others, hard work for many and, sadly, for some couples it's impossible. I knew one in eight couples had difficulty conceiving, so I never assumed I'd fall pregnant easily but of course hoped I would. After eight months of unsuccessful well-timed effort my partner and I went for tests to discover what was going wrong. The problem was sperm antibodies interfering with fertilisation. Each of my eggs needed to be fertilised by being injected with one of his sperm. This would be done via IVF.

The process of IVF is an emotional roller-coaster; exciting and terrifying when you begin a cycle and devastating when it fails. The snorting and injecting of hormones, the blood tests, internals and ultrasounds would be easy if you could be sure you'd be pregnant this time or next time or the time after that. The traumatic part is, you have no idea whether you'll *ever* fall pregnant and if you do, that you won't miscarry.

Looking back, I'm amazed that for our treatment cycles we were so keen to have three fertilised eggs transferred. This meant possible triplets, but also possibly still no pregnancy. Having become so used to not becoming pregnant we wanted to give it the best chance. I've since spoken to many IVF twin mums who chose to transfer two fertilised eggs even after a couple of unsuccessful cycles. Oddly, while doing the cycle, we talked a lot about whether or not I'd be pregnant but barely mentioned twins, let alone triplets. We both knew that a pregnancy after three fertilised eggs have been transferred meant a 20 per cent chance of twins and a five per cent chance of triplets.

I've since learnt that when two good-quality eggs are transferred there is a 25 per cent chance of pregnancy, and with three good-quality eggs, the chance of pregnancy is only increased to 26 per cent. I wish I'd known and been able to weigh up our chances versus the risk of triplets, given the physical, social, emotional and financial consequences.

Having done my second IVF cycle, I found out I was pregnant the day my period was due. My nurse said there was a possibility of more than one baby, as my hormone levels were high but I put that possibility straight out of my mind. Didn't dare to hope. I had an ultrasound four weeks later. Any ultrasound scan done at that stage of a pregnancy shows a tiny little stick with a beating heart, which is what we saw on the screen. One tiny little stick with a heartbeat. Just beautiful. I have a vague memory of the ultrasound technician also mentioning an unviable sac. I was pregnant and happy.

Being determined to know absolutely everything there was to know about my condition meant reading everything I could, so when friends commented on the fact that I was 'showing' I strongly denied it. I knew that a first pregnancy wasn't noticeable until after 12 weeks. There was no way that bulge had anything to do with the baby, I was just eating too much. At six weeks I was desperate to feel some nausea, a physical sign of my precious state. Come on, come on, why don't I feel sick? Am I still pregnant? Then it hit me. I felt sicker than I'd ever felt in my life. I puked all day and all night. For four weeks I lay in bed with a towel and a bucket. The sickness was totally debilitating. My brother came around every day with a cure. The girl in the milkbar said lemonade. His mate's wife used ginger tablets. Dry biscuits, grated apple – I am never, never, never doing this again. Why would anyone ever have a second pregnancy? I lost six kilos and thought back to those earlier weeks when I was begging for that sick feeling.

The other overwhelming feeling during these early days was terror at the prospect of miscarriage, made even worse by the prospect of being unable to fall pregnant again. I was counting down the days till I hit that magical 12 weeks when I could be confident that things might turn out OK.

At 14 weeks, nausea all but gone, it was time to go back to the clinic to check out our baby. The night before the ultrasound I lay in bed thinking about the size of my belly. Maybe there are two babies in there. No, obviously the baby had 'oesophageal atresia', where the foetus can't swallow amniotic fluid so the amniotic fluid builds up causing dangerous problems. That's what's wrong with the baby. I'm way too big. I panicked.

Lying on the table at the clinic I was looking at the screen but couldn't make out a thing. Suddenly the technician said, 'Well, (long pause) there are two babies here.' Silence. Relief. It wasn't a terrible amniotic fluid problem, I wasn't dying and neither was the baby. I laughed and laughed while Tony sat there with a huge grin on his face. Then suddenly I felt horrified. One baby hadn't been there last time. The new baby was tiny. 'It's too small. Quick, measure it. Is it normal? Will it be OK?'

It seemed to take forever to measure the baby but it was within the normal range. Everything looked fine. Relaxed again, we chatted, fell silent then laughed all the way home. We rang our families immediately. Then we rang everyone else. Everyone.

It was after the news had really sunk in that I admitted that since I'd been pregnant, I'd felt intense pangs of jealousy whenever I saw a woman with two children. My mind would wander onto whether I'd need to do IVF again and whether I'd be successful. I had greedy, selfish thoughts of wanting more than one child.

As we digested the news we tried to figure out exactly how difficult our new life was going to be. We knew we were in for hard work but how hard? And what about the pregnancy? What should we expect?

Adjusting to the news

For many, it's great news to hear you're having two babies. But for just as many, it means a big adjustment. Many parents experience negative feelings at first. Most women's feelings swing from one extreme to the other during pregnancy. The extra hormones caused by a twin pregnancy mean these swings may be more dramatic. Regardless of whether your pregnancy makes you delighted, depressed or somewhere in between you will probably experience highs and lows.

Psychological or emotional concerns
- You might be concerned about having two babies at once.
- You may have been counting on having only one or one more baby.
- You may fear losing one or both babies.
- You may feel that people are ready to discuss the positives but are unable to deal with the negative emotions about your pregnancy.
- You may feel isolated from those you know who are having one baby at a time.
- You may be a single parent and find the idea overwhelming.
- You may be concerned that your other children's needs might be neglected because of the demands of two small babies.
- You may be concerned about the emotional strain on your relationship.
- Feeding two babies may be a mind-boggling concept.

Physical challenges
- Twin pregnancies are more physically demanding and are considered more risky.
- You may need more medical intervention during your pregnancy and labour.
- Twins are more likely to be born pre-term or small – 37 weeks is often considered full term.
- Your babies may need to be in special care and so they will spend more time in hospital.
- You will obviously be larger than you would be with one baby and this will slow you down in getting ready for your babies. (The chance of spending some time unable to do much or on strict bed rest is more common with twin pregnancies.)
- Older couples expecting twins may be worried about meeting the physical demands of two babies.

Financial issues
- You may have to leave work earlier, as the physical strain may be greater than with a single pregnancy.

- You may have timed this pregnancy based on the cost of one baby and be concerned about meeting the costs of two.
- You may need to pay for help around the house.
- Your plans to return to work may be altered when you find it's two babies, not one – childcare for two (or more) can be more expensive.
- You may have to move to a larger home.
- You may need a bigger car.

Being shocked or devastated is a healthy reaction to such big news, as is an overwhelming feeling of joy. Feelings of inadequacy are also a natural response. Some women hope to miscarry one baby or even both. If you are concerned about your emotional response or feel you need more than a friend to talk to, get help straightaway. Your GP can refer you to a counsellor. There is a comprehensive list of phone numbers you can call for help in the back of this book.

Remember many people have 'bad' thoughts as a natural response to big news. Don't be hard on yourself.

Pregnancy after fertility treatment

ANOTHER MUM SAYS   'My two-year-old twins are a complete joy. They're great friends and my husband and I are so proud of them.'

The idea that fertility treatment and programs increase your chances of conceiving twins often appeals to couples who have spent years unsuccessfully trying to conceive. The Australian Bureau of Statistics states that 20 per cent of multiple births in Australia result from fertility programs.

Some couples feel that they are bound to have twins because they are using fertility treatment and are disappointed when they have an ultrasound showing a single baby. Others are relieved to be having just twins, not triplets or more, after ovulation induction or a three-egg transfer.

Often for couples using IVF, GIFT or other fertility treatments, the desire for a baby is so strong that when they learn they are expecting twins they feel they should be over the moon. It's not always that simple.

Infertility is a social problem as well as a medical one. It can still be surrounded by secrecy and taboo even though it is incredibly common.

Some statistics say that one in six Australian couples have difficulty conceiving. Complete strangers will ask mothers of twins whether they took fertility drugs or whether their babies are 'natural'. Try not to get annoyed. Some people are insensitive or nosey but a percentage of these people will be approaching you because they are unable to get pregnant themselves and may prefer to talk about it with a stranger. The experience is isolating and can cause intense feelings in both partners, who often feel they are 'going crazy' and are desperate to discuss their feelings with those who can reassure them they are 'normal'.

There is no increased risk for postnatal depression after fertility treatment. Those who do have difficulty find it is because those around them believe they shouldn't, because their dream of having children has finally been realised. This denial can reinforce feelings of inadequacy and also prevent those with problems from talking or seeking help.

Another positive outcome of fertility treatment is that you become more confident about asking for what you want and are more used to medical procedures and intervention.

> (ANOTHER MUM SAYS)   'I was counting my blessings. To fall pregnant with one baby using IVF was such great news. When they found an extra baby at my second ultrasound I felt like I'd won Tattslotto.'

Emotional responses

Emotional issues arising from medically assisted conception of twins may include:

- A pregnancy that's been difficult to achieve may make you more fearful of something going wrong. Talk to your doctor or obstetrician about your concerns. Talking with friends or family may also help.
- You may not have expected to fall pregnant at all, let alone with twins, so you may be upset when fertility treatment is finally successful.
- You may be concerned about the higher risk of caesarean section – 53 per cent of twin pregnancies after conception using reproductive technologies, according to ACCESS Australia's National Infertility Network.
- You may be concerned about the increased risk of prematurity with a twin IVF pregnancy. For unknown reasons IVF pregnancies are more likely to be pre-term than spontaneously conceived pregnancies.

- You may feel you 'shouldn't' complain about fears or discomforts during your pregnancy because you're 'lucky' to be pregnant and your doctor and family are so delighted.
- You may resent that the possibility and implications of a twin pregnancy and of raising twins was skimmed over in fertility treatment counselling.
- You may be used to a lot of attention, being prodded, pushed, blood tests, everything – then suddenly when you're pregnant with twins, the IVF team has finished with you and you're waiting to see a doctor or obstetrician who doesn't need to spend much time with you. You may feel abandoned while also feeling precious.
- IVF pregnancies can be considered high-risk.

ANOTHER MUM SAYS 'By the time my IVF worked, I'd had four treatments and I'd just come to terms with being child-free and had planned my whole new independent life. My doctor said to me 'It's worked, Mum' and suddenly I was expecting twins. I felt my life had come to a complete end. Then I felt so guilty for not appreciating this more. I didn't bond with my babies until way into the pregnancy when I could feel them kicking. I started to allow myself to love them.'

ANOTHER MUM SAYS 'I sometimes feel that because we went through so much to conceive our twins we focus on the great things about having twins and just deal with the difficulties. There are times when I feel that I would like to be a normal first time mother going through what I term the honeymoon period of parenting. That is just having one child to devote my time to, not jumping in at the deep end like you do with twins. Some people say to me that I should be glad that it is all over in one hit, instant family. I don't feel this way. I love parenting and I don't want it all to be over in one hit.

I am very open about the boys being conceived through IVF. I don't think it is anything to be ashamed of. We are very grateful that the technology was available to help us.

Egg transfer

The number of eggs to transfer in one cycle is a hot research topic at the moment. There is a world-wide trend to transfer only two embryos and the aim is to get that down to one. Some Australian IVF clinics are currently conducting trials where one embryo (rather than two) will be transferred and with improved techniques it is hoped there will be no difference in the pregnancy rate. Current health and community services are ill-equipped to support families with a multiple birth. Multiple births also need additional hospital support, with greater likelihood of pre-term birth.

Foetal reduction

Foetal reduction is the practice of reducing the number of embryos in the uterus. Those with triplets or higher order multiples may decide for many reasons to reduce the number of embryos. This can be a very difficult option and you may need to think it through carefully and discuss it with your doctor and a psychologist to reach the decision that is right for you.

> ANOTHER MUM SAYS   'I was devastated when I found out we were having triplets. We had no money and no family to call on. We felt twins were more than we could cope with. Which baby did they choose to inject and why? I felt and still feel it was a cruel thing to do but believe I was choosing between a family being completely blown apart and a family that might just make it. We haven't told any of our friends about it and will never tell the boys. It's a sad, private corner of our hearts.'

Twin types

The term 'twins' comes from the ancient German word 'twin' or 'twine' meaning 'two together'. There are many types of twins. The two obvious categories are Monozygotic (MZ) or identical, and Dizygotic (DZ) or fraternal, but there are some surprising sub-types.

Monozygotic (MZ) twins

An MZ twin pregnancy starts in the same way as a singleton pregnancy where a single egg is fertilised by a single sperm. The cells of the fertilised egg (zygote) start to divide and multiply in the usual way. The zygote divides one extra time and splits apart, creating two separate but genetically identical zygotes. MZ twins are often referred to as 'identical'. They look very similar but they are two different people.

It is not known why this split occurs but it is the subject of ongoing research.

MZ twins can have two placentas if the zygote or egg splits within three days of conception; otherwise they share one placenta. They can be different sizes if intra-uterine nourishment has been different. Despite having the same genes, identical twins have different fingerprints. This is due to environmental factors both in and out of the uterus.

There's as much chance of having a pair of girls as a pair of boys. Having MZ twins does not run in the family, it can happen to anybody.

Mirror-image twins: Twenty-five per cent of MZ twins are mirror-image. Their physical features are on opposite sides of their bodies. For example, one will be left-handed, and the other right-handed. Also the hair crown grows in opposite directions and birthmarks and moles appear on opposite sides. Sometimes their internal organs are also on opposite sides.

Conjoined twins: When the division of the zygote occurs late the zygote doesn't always split completely and conjoined twins result. Conjoined twins can be connected at any point on their body but both will be connected at the same place.

Conjoined twins used to be known as Siamese twins, from the country of origin of Chang and Eng Bunker, conjoined twins who were born in 1811 in Thailand, known then as Siam. Chang and Eng were joined at the chest. They married two American sisters, and one had ten children and the other had twelve. They divided their time between their two family homes. One was a drinker while the other abstained. They died at the age of 63 within sixteen hours of each other after Chang's drinking contributed to liver failure.

Conjoined twins occur in one in 100 000 births or one in 200 pairs of MZ twins. They share placentas and membranes and can share body parts and organs. They are usually identified by ultrasound early in the pregnancy. Recently several pairs of conjoined twins have been successfully separated.

Dizygotic (DZ) twins

DZ twins are often called 'fraternal' twins. They are conceived when the mother produces two separate eggs in the same monthly cycle or during IVF when more than one embryo is transferred to the mother's uterus; each egg is fertilised by a separate sperm and they become two separate babies. They will only look as alike as any pair of siblings, often with a family resemblance but quite different.

DZ twins always have separate placentas but sometimes these fuse together, giving the appearance of one placenta. When looking at the ultrasound or at the actual placenta it can be impossible to tell whether two placentas have fused or whether there is a shared placenta.

DZ twins can be the result of superfecundation, where the conceptions take place on two separate occasions, over a couple of days of fertility. One foetus can be a few days older and consequently slightly more developed. This also means the possibility of fraternal twins with the same mother but two different fathers if sperm from two different men fertilise an egg each.

Fraternal twins run in families through the maternal side as some women have a genetic tendency to ovulate more than one egg at time. If twins are in the father's family, this will not increase the mother's chances of having twins. However, men from families with fraternal twins can carry the gene and pass it on to their daughters, who could then conceive twins, which is why twins are thought to skip a generation.

Women who have had three or more children are also more likely to conceive fraternal twins. Fraternal twins are also more common in mothers aged 34–39, as women tend to ovulate more erratically during these years.

Half of all fraternal twins are boy/girl pairs, one quarter are boy/boy and one quarter girl/girl.

Half-identical twins (a third type of twin)
There is some debate about whether 'half-identical' twins exist. This is when the egg splits *before* fertilisation and each half is fertilised by two different sperm. The twins have identical genes from the mother but not from the father. These two sperm could be from the same father, or two different fathers.

How to tell if your twins are MZ or DZ
Some parents have no real desire to know whether their twins are officially 'identical'. Examining the placenta and the membrane alone is not a reliable way to determine if your babies are MZ or DZ twins.

Working it out is usually straightforward. If other people have trouble telling them apart, then they're probably MZ. Knowing helps you work out your likelihood of having twins again in the future and may be of some medical benefit. You will also need to be sure if the twins are participating in twin study research.

If your babies are a boy/girl pair, if they have different eye and hair colour or different blood types, they're DZ. But twins with the same gender, colouring and blood type can still be DZ. Microscopic examination of the placenta will give an indication, but only DNA testing the babies will give you a conclusive answer.

If your children were helped into the world through assisted reproduction technologies, there is still the possibility that they are MZ.

Twin facts

Over 4000 Australian and over 850 New Zealand families will have twins in 2005. Throughout the developed world the rate of multiple births is increasing. Australian statistics reflect this.

YEAR	FREQUENCY
1980	one in 100 births
1990	one in 84 births
2000	one in 65 births
2002	one in 60 births

Source: Australian Bureau of Statistics

The frequency of twins is increasing due to three main factors.

Firstly, improved medical intervention and postnatal care means twins have an increasing survival rate. Secondly, IVF, GIFT, Clomid (a fertility drug) and other fertility treatments can increase the likelihood of multiple births. Third, couples are delaying their families and women between the ages of 34 and 39 are more likely to conceive DZ (non-identical) twins.

A collaborative study by La Trobe University, the Royal Women's Hospital in Melbourne and the TVW Telethon Institute for Child Health Research in Perth found that women who take folate supplements may also have an increased chance of conceiving and bearing twins. It is current practice for health professionals to recommend that women planning to conceive, and in the first trimester of pregnancy, to take a folic acid supplement to reduce the likelihood of neural tube defects such as spina bifida. This study found a higher incidence of twins born to women with high folate levels. It reported the possibility that each twin became more 'viable' with the mother's higher folate level.

> ### VANISHING TWIN SYNDROME
>
> This is when one twin dies in utero and is reabsorbed into the placenta. This happens before 12 weeks and is more common in the first eight weeks of pregnancy. It is thought to happen in one out of every five twin conceptions. Many mothers do not have an ultrasound before 12 weeks but modern techniques mean we are often scanned earlier are more likely to be aware of this pregnancy loss. One baby can disappear with or without vaginal bleeding and this may not be known until the next ultrasound.
>
> Vanishing twin syndrome can be devastating. Parents are not alone in their suffering, other family and friends will also feel the loss. There are support groups are available where you can meet and talk with others who share your experience. See Resources, pages 340–47 for a list of support groups.

There are some confused theories but some interesting facts are:

- About one in 12 pregnancies begin as twins, but in many only one baby thrives.
- Africans have the highest incidence of twinning, followed by Europeans, Mexicans then Asians.
- Boy/girl twin pairs cannot be identical.
- Parenting twins is very different from parenting two babies close in age.
- Twenty per cent of twins are left-handed while less than ten per cent of the general population are left-handed.
- Some twins claim to share a psychic connection, even feeling phantom pain when the other is hurt.
- Twins have been known to develop a language that only they understand. This process is known as cryptophasia.
- One out of three sets of twins in Australia and New Zealand is identical.
- Identical twins do not run in families.
- MZ twins are thought to be more common in IVF than in the general population. An IVF fertilised egg seems more likely to split than a naturally conceived fertilised egg.
- Parents of MZ twins usually do not get them confused, although everybody else does.

- MZ twins reared apart in very different families tend to get the same score on IQ tests.
- Some MZ twins reared apart have had major life events like the death of a child or mental illness of a spouse at the same time.
- The less time MZ twins spend together the more similar they become.
- DZ twins can run in families but do not necessarily 'skip' a generation.
- If you've spontaneously conceived one set of DZ twins, you have a one in four chance of conceiving twins in a subsequent pregnancy.
- There is current research trying both to prove and disprove the idea that DZ twins may be genetically closer than siblings.

Twins are good for your health

Health researchers recognise that twins and their families are very special people. The similarities and differences that make twins interesting to everyone are the very things that enable researchers to study the relative impact of genetic and environmental factors on health and the treatment and prevention of disease.

If MZ pairs are more similar for a characteristic than DZ pairs, especially if the MZ pairs are reared apart, then it is likely that genetic factors are playing a role in that characteristic. The involvement of twins in genetic research is a vital contribution to search for answers to the profound questions posed by this hot topic.

The Australian Twin Registry is a data base that uses twins in research. It helps researchers contact twins who might be interested in taking part in approved research projects. The Twin Registry is funded by the federal government. Participation is voluntary and approved projects satisfy stringent ethical guidelines. Steve and Mark Waugh, twin brothers well known for their achievements in cricket, are co-patrons of the Australian Twin Registry.

Since 1980, more than 30000 pairs of Australian twins have joined the Australian Twin Registry, making it the largest volunteer registry of its kind in the world. This is about twenty per cent of all twins living in Australia. Contact details for the registry are supplied on page 340).

**FRIGHTENING FACTS FROM THE
GUINNESS BOOK OF RECORDS**

- Mary Jones of the UK, who died in 1899, gave birth to
  15 sets of twins.
- Anna Steynvaait of South Africa gave birth to 2 sets of twins in
  12 months.
- Barbara Zula of South Africa had 6 sets of twins in 6 years (1967–73).

Surviving the news

One of the things that helps most during a twin pregnancy is meeting other sane and happy parents of twins. Watching them interact with their children, talking with them about how special their twins are and just seeing them cope is reassuring. You will probably be playing 'spot-the-twins' nearly every time you go out and wondering why you hadn't previously noticed them. Don't be afraid to stop twin parents in the street and ask them questions. Most parents of twins are delighted to talk with others expecting twins.

The Australian Multiple Birth Association (AMBA) and the New Zealand Multiple Births Association (NZMBA) offer a variety of services and networks. AMBA is a voluntary organisation run by busy parents of multiples with membership of 5000 families. Every Australian state and territory has a branch which offers a variety of services and networks for parents of twins. You can use the AMBA newsletter to contact others in your situation. Contact details for your local branch of AMBA and NZMBA are given in Resources (see pages 340–347). Some of the resources AMBA and NZMBA makes available to members include:

- antenatal nights
- hospital and home visits
- pram hire
- social events with other families
- playgroups
- informative leaflets and publications
- library of twin books and other resources
- contacts for specialist support groups such as breastfeeding, bereavement, pre-term babies, disabilities

Remember that there is no 'right' way to feel about having twins. Talk, talk, talk to anyone who'll listen. People will be interested, and you'll sort out your own feelings by talking about them. Find out as much as you can. There are web sites with chat rooms about twins (see Resources, pages 340–47), and you can visit your local maternal child health care centre, introduce yourself and ask for any information on parenting twins. They should have an AMBA or NZMBA video available for you to borrow.

From the minute you find out that you're having twins, start looking after your body with a healthy diet, some exercise and plenty of rest. Visit a physiotherapist dealing in women's health for advice on looking after your changing body. Sort out your finances. Pull all your income and expense records out of the bottom drawer and organise yourself or take them to a financial adviser. Financial advisers are not just for people with lots of money but for those without enough as well. If your income is low enough, you may be able to see one free of charge through your local council. Contact the Family Assistance Office (see Resources, pages 340–47) to see what payments you are eligible to receive.

Talk with your partner, speculate on what your new life may be like and make some plans for coping while you are both clear-headed and sleeping well. And start thinking about who's going to be helpful, how they'd like to help, what help you need and schedule them in.

FAMOUS TWINS

- B1 and B2 (ABC's Bananas in Pyjamas)
- Bob the Builder (BBC Children's TV character) has a twin brother, Tom
- Senator Bob Brown (Australian Greens Senator) has a twin sister
- Steve and Mark Waugh (Australian cricketing legends) are twins
- Vince Colosimo (Australian actor) is a twin
- Isabella Rossellini (actress) is a twin
- Robin and Maurice Gibb from The Bee Gees are twins
- Elvis Presley was a twin (his brother, Jesse, was stillborn)
- Alanis Morissette (pop singer) has a twin brother, Wade
- Jerry Hall (model and actor) has a twin sister
- Mary-Kate and Ashley Olsen (celebrities) are twins
- Kiefer Sutherland (actor and son of Donald) is a twin
- Liberace (pianist), had a twin who died at birth

TIPS FOR SURVIVING THE NEWS THAT IT'S TWINS

- Enjoy the attention of family, friends and acquaintances.
- Talk about how you are feeling to anyone who will listen.
- Start organising your finances.
- Start looking after your body.
- Contact AMBA or NZMBA.

TIPS FOR PARTNERS

- Prepare yourself to be much more hands-on than if there was one baby.
- Listen to and talk with your partner.
- Find out as much as you can about twins.
- Be involved in all the medical appointments from the start.
- Make her feel special and pampered. It's hard work being pregnant with twins.

Turkey platters and toilet bowls

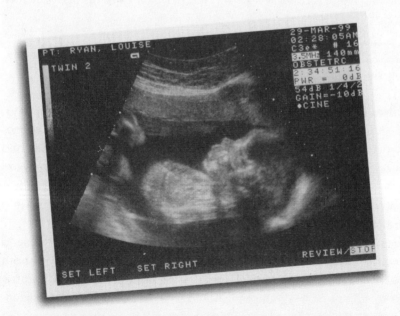

PT: RYAN, LOUISE
TWIN 2
29-MAR-99
02:28:05AM
C3e* # 16
3.5MHz 140mm
OBSTETRC
2:34:51 16
PWR = 0dB
54dB 1/4/2
GAIN=-10dB
*CINE
REVIEW/STOP
SET LEFT   SET RIGHT

PREGNANCY

PREGNANCY: OUR STORIES

There are many similarities between a single-baby pregnancy and a twin pregnancy but there are important physical differences. Twin pregnancies are considered higher risk but many of the difficulties can be managed and some can be prevented. Looking after yourself by eating and resting properly are the two main ways you can actively support your health and the health of your babies.

The possible discomforts of a pregnancy can arrive earlier and be more extreme with twins than in a single-baby pregnancy. By knowing what to watch out for and how to look after yourself, you're giving your babies the best possible start.

Recognising the warning signs and symptoms can mean seeking earlier treatment.

Twins are likely to be born earlier than single babies. The average twin gestation is 36 weeks rather than 40. The exact reason isn't known but the uterus being stretched to its limits and the weight of the twin pregnancy may signal to the body that it's time for labour to start. You may be aiming for a particular date but stay flexible. Thirty-five per cent of twins arrive before 35 weeks and ten per cent of twins arrive before 31 weeks.

ANOTHER MUM SAYS   'I'll be able to balance the turkey platter on my belly by Christmas day if I keep growing at this rate!'

Katrina: When I was told I was having twins, I cried for the first four days. Day five was my birthday. I spent the evening eating my birthday chocolates and telling my friends the 'bad' news over the phone. I finally had the strength to call my mother. She said it was a double blessing. Mum reminded me that my godmother had identical twin boys after her two daughters. She's sane, she has a career and her children are great fun and well balanced.

My GP wrote 'anxious' on my medical card for reference. My husband was worried, and didn't know how to deal with me. He was happy about the news. He was very proud of himself – he figured his sperm had the power to split eggs. He thought I should snap out of it, accept the situation and soldier on. I agreed with him, but didn't know how to.

At my first ultrasound there was concern that there might not be a membrane dividing the babies into two sacs. This meant the umbilical cords could become tangled. I quickly started to learn why twin pregnancies are more risky. A membrane showed up on later scans, but it was so 'fine' it indicated that our twins were probably identical.

I had been really tired through my first trimester, all I did was work shorter hours and operate the remote control from the couch. The 12 week turnaround was instant. I suddenly had energy to burn and was feeling great. From around 30 weeks it was back to life on the couch. It was summer and my feet and ankles were elephantine. My belly was big, but not as big as I expected it to be.

I rang our local Australian Multiple Birth Association contact and was greeted with warmth and friendship and invited to the Christmas party to meet some twins and parents. It was a very busy and noisy party. 'It's as hard as you want it to be,' I was told. At first I found this comforting. Later I realised that comment had been aimed at keeping me in a positive frame of mind. I wasn't feeling up to it.

Then slowly I began to feel a special buzz. Twins came out of the woodwork. Mine wasn't just another office pregnancy. 'You never do things by half', 'twins are only blessed on those who can cope.' I was amazed by people's generosity. Their confidence that I was strong enough started to rub off on me. I began to be able to laugh while I told people about my 'bad luck'. I had no shame in telling people that I didn't want twins. Who in their right mind would want more than one baby at a time?

I gradually started to realise that my babies will share things that no one else will ever know or understand. Reading stories of other mothers with twins, hearing their happiness, learning how special twins are, the bond that they have. Most of us spend our lives searching for someone who knows us intimately and understands us. I saw it as my job to nurture their individuality while not ignoring their twinship. But at the same time I felt jealous that they would have this bond while I must sacrifice everything.

I started reading on the Internet about twin-to-twin transfusion and was frightened by the extra risks in a twin pregnancy. My obstetrician told me not to rush out and buy double everything just yet. It was a warning – don't start getting your hopes up, dearie. Just when I had started getting used to the idea.

At work I went from being the first person in and last to leave, to the opposite. I also had the longest lunch break, taking full advantage of the bed in the sick bay. I recognised that I didn't have to do everything myself and learnt to delegate and reduce my expectations of myself. I achieved almost as much and still managed to look after myself.

We went to the antenatal classes at our local hospital. The class was all one-baby specific and was irrelevant to me. We kept going because they taught relaxation techniques, gave us a hospital tour and I met other prospective mums. The midwife said one thing that made me feel good. She said, with twins, labour is often faster and less strenuous. The pressure of two babies means you can be three centimetres or more dilated and not even know it. It helps speed things along. At last, a plus!

So much of my energy was consumed with the babies' growth. My husband took over the household so that I could take every opportunity to rest. We started going into their 'room' and picturing the babies in it. We were looking forward to meeting our babies so we could tell them how much we loved them. I felt both joy and fear – how would we cope?

Reaching that 33-week mark was an important milestone for us. If the babies arrived before then they would need intensive care, which was not available in the town where we lived. It would mean transfer by ambulance or helicopter hundreds of kilometres from home. I stopped work at 33 weeks to give myself a bit of time at home in case they came early. I barely made it that far and my physical and emotional capacity was pushed to the limits. I loved my job, but it was a relief to leave. Office politics had become so meaningless. I needed to focus on the task ahead.

Louise: From 14 weeks until the end I had a perfect pregnancy. In fact I felt better than I'd ever felt. I was still nervous about everything being OK but felt happy, happy, happy. I was filled with energy. I told anyone who'd listen that I was having twins. Yes, that's right, TWO babies. In here! Happily whipping my shirt up for all to see. I found it hard to believe it was possible to grow two babies in that space. It became more of a reality when my organs seemed to be struggling for room.

I accosted families with twins whenever I saw them. What's it like? Tell me something. What do I need to know? Everyone was interested in the babies, there was a novelty value attached to twins.

I threw up every morning, including the day the girls were born but this just became ritual. I could time it so it was simply a part of the day. Every day I ate an entire pineapple and drank two litres of milk. At six months I started to topple over. Just walking along I'd lose my balance and fall. My centre of gravity had changed. The last time I fell I ended up with scraped elbows and knees, quite a mess, so I ditched all my shoes and put on my runners and left them on for the next three months. No one complained about anything when they knew there were two babies. Besides it was practical, comfortable and safe.

I loved visiting my doctor but was always a bit nervous until the stethoscope picked up the sound of those two beating hearts. One of my babies was quite a bit smaller than average so I was always concerned to see that everything was OK. I judged the size of the small baby by comparing the two and hoping each visit that the gap was closing. It stayed much the same until their birth. I also loved the feel of the babies moving around. They moved differently, it was easy to tell which was which and when they were changing places or somersaulting. Often I could see an elbow or knee move across my belly.

One night at about 26 weeks I was cooking dinner and got an electric shock when I was lighting the stove. It wasn't a big shock but it gave me a huge fright – I wasn't sure how it would affect the babies. Would it have shocked their little hearts into stopping? Does amniotic fluid act as a conductor? Tony rang the hospital and they said to come in immediately. I sat waiting to feel those kicks. Nothing. It was a long, long half-hour waiting to see a doctor, then finding their heartbeats took forever. Tony was as white as a sheet. It was such a relief when they finally found them, those little boom-booms.

I got irritated when other people didn't recognise the physical stress a twin pregnancy puts on your body. How tired you get. I just wanted to sit down. I was carrying 25 kilos. Imagine carrying five big bags of potatoes around with you everywhere you went. That's hard work. I even had to take my five bags of potatoes to bed with me and bring them to the loo a few times a night.

I decided I would like to work every morning and found someone to do the afternoons who would also take over full-time for my maternity leave period. I divided the work so the tasks I did were the lighter ones. My boss was delighted as it meant all the planning and organising was done. At 28 weeks I felt like I should stop work completely but my doctor seemed to see no need and we were short of money so I soldiered on. I would never have continued to work if I'd known that fatigue, standing for too long and carrying things can trigger pre-term labour. My instincts were telling me to rest and I wasn't listening. I worked until I was 33 weeks pregnant.

As I hadn't had a vaginal birth before, my doctor wanted to organise an elective caesarean. He felt it was too risky to deliver these babies vaginally. He said he wouldn't let his wife do it and couldn't do it for me. He would refer me to someone else if I wanted to plan a vaginal delivery. I was keen to stick with him as he'd transferred my tiny IVF fertilised eggs and it seemed right that he'd be the one to take them out again. I was also keen to avoid risk. I just wanted healthy babies and I trusted him completely to look after us all.

I spent a lot of time trying to imagine and prepare for two babies but my imagination couldn't stretch beyond the birth and arriving home. I made and froze mountains of bolognaise sauce, casseroles and soups – about 40 meals to see us through that first month.

At 25 weeks I got to know four other girls expecting twins at the same time. We met through our local multiple-birth group so lived quite near each other. We continued to catch up every couple of weeks, comparing tummies, aches, pains, itches, fears and plans. One by one we delivered: vaginal births, caesareans, blood transfusions, epidurals, spinal blocks, no drugs at all, premmie babies, small-for-dates babies, tube-fed babies, babies in isolettes, girls, boys, both. Five mums, ten babies and fifteen different stories.

Development of a twin pregnancy

Through your pregnancy, visualise the size and development of your babies. It may help you to slow down, eat well, drink water and rest when you see how much work your body is doing building these two new lives.

TWINS' HEAD SIZE IN UTERO

12 weeks – 2 grapes	28 weeks – 2 lemons
16 weeks – 2 apricots	32 weeks – 2 large oranges
20 weeks – 2 eggs	36 weeks – 2 grapefruit
24 weeks – 2 tangerines	40 weeks – 2 small canteloupes (rockmelons)

Week 1   Your period begins.

Week 2   The lining of the uterus thickens to prepare for a possible pregnancy, one or more eggs are released from the ovary and are
fertilised by sperm as they move down the fallopian tube to the
uterus.

Week 3   The eggs are implanted in your endometrium (the lining of your
uterus) where they are nourished through the blood supply.

Week 4   Your babies' placenta or placentas grow deeper into the
endometrium. Your blood supply to the placentas ensures that
nutrients are taken to the babies while their waste is taken away.

Week 5   The babies' spinal cords, nervous systems, hearts and circulation
are all developing. Your blood supply supports them so they are
no longer dependent on the nutrients from the eggs. By the end of
this week both umbilical cords have been formed.

Week 6   Your babies' hearts begin to beat. There may be visible signs that
their arms and legs are beginning to form.

Weeks 7 & 8   The babies look more C-shaped, their eyes develop and their fingers and outer ears start to take shape, followed closely by their
toes.

Weeks 9 & 10   Your babies' fingers, toes and ears become more developed, so
they now look distinctly human. By the end of the 10th week all
their major organs are formed. The amniotic sac(s) have developed between the babies and the placenta(s) and have filled with
fluid. The babies float in their sacs, protected in a perfect environment.

Month 3   Your babies' faces take shape and eyes are in place. Their brains
have been growing quickly. Their genitals are clearly developed
and their arms are in proportion to their bodies with legs following
closely behind.

Months 4 & 5   Each baby is growing rapidly longer, they are half the size they will
be at full term. You can see their hair and eyebrows and feel their
kicks.

Months 6 & 7   Their skin is red and wrinkly and their respiratory and nervous systems are developing quickly but are not yet able to function outside the uterus, without help.

Months 8 & 9   Your babies' heads are putting on weight and becoming more
rounded.

Eating – what to eat and how much

What you eat has a direct influence on the development and birth weight of your babies. What they weigh at birth is shown to have an impact on their future health. Heavier babies are more likely to become healthier children and adults. Healthy eating while you're pregnant may reduce the chances of your babies being born too early.

Your babies take the nutrients they need first so you will suffer if you don't eat properly during your pregnancy. A twin pregnancy requires more food than what you've been used to eating. Gaining weight eating the right foods helps to keep you healthy and your babies growing well.

> Eat 3 meals per day plus 4 substantial snacks.
> Eat every 2 hours if you are struggling to eat the right volume of food.
> Don't wait until you're hungry.

The Department of Nutrition & Dietetics at the Royal Women's Hospital, Melbourne, suggests that by eating the serves in the chart below, your calories will be spread across a range of foods.

DAIRY: 4–5 SERVES PER DAY
1 serve = 1 cup milk
1 serve = 1 cup cottage cheese
1 serve = 1 slice hard cheese (35 g)
1 serve = 1 tub yoghurt

MEAT, FISH, POULTRY OR PROTEIN SUBSTITUTES: 2 SERVES PER DAY
1 serve = 100 g lean meat or chicken
1 serve = 200 g fish
1 serve = 1 cup cooked beans
1 serve = 2 eggs

BREAD AND CEREALS: 4–6 SERVES PER DAY
1 serve = 1 slice of bread
1 serve = $^3/4$ cup of cereal
1 serve = $^1/2$ cup of rice or pasta
1 serve = two wholemeal biscuits

FRUIT AND VEGETABLES: AT LEAST 6–8 SERVES PER DAY

1 serve = 1/3 cup of vegies

1 serve = 1 piece of fruit

1 serve = glass of orange juice

Make sure one serve is a dark-green, leafy vegetable –
broccoli, spinach etc.

OIL, BUTTER OR CREAM PER DAY:

1–2 tablespoons

SUGAR:

Eat least and enjoy as a treat

(ANOTHER MUM SAYS)   'I was hungry the whole time. I found myself
having to get up at 4 a.m. to eat then go back to bed.'

Water

Drinking two litres of water a day prevents dehydration. If drinking this much water is difficult, try adding a splash of fruit juice. Drinking water also lowers the risk of urinary tract infections, which can also lead to pre-term labour. Your babies require a lot of amniotic fluid and you need to avoid headaches and constipation. You should be peeing at least two hourly and your pee should be almost clear in colour. If you're not peeing regularly or the pee appears a concentrated yellow colour, drink more water.

Folic acid

In twin pregnancies mothers are recommended to continue taking at least 400 micrograms of folic acid a day from either food or supplements during the first 12 weeks of pregnancy to lower your chances of having babies with neural tube defects like spina bifida. Foods rich in folic acid include citrus fruits, sardines, baked beans and green leafy vegetables.

Vegetarians

A vegetarian diet can meet the needs of pregnancy if care is taken to include adequate protein, iron, vitamin B 12 and foods containing calcium. Your increased protein requirements in pregnancy are usually met by the extra calories from more foods. Milk, cheese, eggs, nuts, seeds, pulses, cereals and soya products like tofu are all good protein sources. Because iron is not absorbed as well from these foods as it is from meat, vegetarians also need to eat plenty of other foods containing iron.

Calcium

Extra calcium is required during pregnancy, to help the babies' bones develop. Good sources of calcium include milk, tofu, cheese, yoghurt, soy and tinned fish with bones, e.g. salmon, sardines.

Vitamins

Vitamin D assists in calcium absorption and can be obtained from sunlight, margarine and dairy products. Adequate amounts of dairy products, meat and eggs are the best sources of vitamin B12 which is essential to the growth and development of your baby. Your need for iron is increased and good sources of absorbable iron include meat, chicken, fish and breakfast cereals with iron added.

It's even more important to consume vitamin C with your iron rich foods to assist absorption. Fresh fruit and vegetables contain vitamin C. An overwhelming desire to eat dirt, chalk, ice or paper while pregnant can indicate an iron deficiency. If the craving hits, speak with your doctor.

If you feel your diet is lacking at all, speak with your medical advisers before taking any vitamins or multi-vitamins. Large amounts of vitamin A aren't good for your babies. Avoid eating liver and liver products such as pâté which contain the animal form of vitamin A.

Foods to avoid

It's best to avoid foods with high listeria potential while you're pregnant. Listeria is an illness caught from eating foods infected with listeriosis. Symptons may include fever, headaches, tiredness, aches and pains or gastro. Listeria can cause miscarriage and pre-term birth.

The foods to avoid are:
- raw fish including sushi, raw or under-cooked meat like rare steak, cold cooked chicken or processed meat like pâté, frankfurts, prosciutto, salami and devon/fritz.
- soft cheeses or cheese like camembert, brie, and feta, mould-ripened cheeses like blue cheese and unpasteurised cheeses made from goats' and sheep's milk should also be avoided, along with soft serve ice-cream.

- pre-prepared salads, raw or soft eggs, including mousse, homemade ice cream and fresh mayonnaise which also have high listeria potential.
- Toxoplasmosis can be contracted from contact with cat poo. Get someone else to empty your cat tray or wear gloves and wash your hands thoroughly if you must do it yourself. Always wear gloves when gardening. Toxoplasmosis can cause miscarriage, pre-term birth and foetal death.

Alcohol

The latest expert advice is to abstain from alcohol which has the potential to cause foetal alcohol syndrome. Small amounts of alcohol are unlikely to have a harmful effect but there is no safe lower limit.

Smoking

Smoking can cause pre-term labour and can also cause babies to have a low birth weight and a higher incidence of respiratory problems. If those around you are smoking, send them outside.

Caffeine

Some research has found that large amounts of caffeine may be harmful in pregnancy. Avoid energy drinks that contain caffeine. Both decaffeinated coffee and dandelion tea can look and smell like the real thing so you could give them a try. Four to five cups of tea a day are fine and three to four cups of weak coffee – not brewed.

Medicines and tablets

During pregnancy and breastfeeding, over-the-counter medicines and tablets (including cold and flu type tablets) shouldn't be taken unless prescribed by your doctor, as they could harm your babies. Seek advice before taking any medicines. If you need pain relief, use paracetamol in the recommended dosage rather than aspirin. Aspirin can cause bleeding problems in pregnancy.

Body shape and size

Women pregnant with twins need to have a steady, healthy weight gain. Your weight gain in early pregnancy influences your babies' rate of growth throughout the rest of the pregnancy. Hormonal changes give your body an opportunity to store some fat and nutrients to use if necessary during the second half of your pregnancy. For some women it's difficult to eat much later in the pregnancy when your babies are squashing your stomach and intestines.

Gaining up to 25 kilos is normal in a twin pregnancy. If you were large prior to your pregnancy, you may be encouraged to gain around 16 kilos. Your weight should increase at one to three kilos per month. Steady weight gain is best. Be wary of a sudden increase in your weight, as it can be linked to pre-eclampsia or gestational diabetes (see pages 51–54).

You'll lose most of the weight you've gained when the babies are born but you'll probably still have loose skin and a pot belly. The pot belly is often from excess fluid that you'll pee and sweat out in the first week after the birth. While a pot belly is not harmful – all women have them after a baby – it can be reduced by gentle exercise such as sit-ups, which can also strengthen your back after birth.

Some fluid retention is normal. You may notice that your rings become a little tighter or your ankles are swollen at the end of the day. Make sure that your fluid retention is not a sign of pre-eclampsia (see pages 53–54).

Maternity bras

Get your maternity bra properly fitted early. Wearing underwire bras while you're pregnant can lead to mastitis and a comfortable bra will change your life.

Sex

Intercourse, orgasm and breast stimulation can help to bring on labour. Because twins are at greater risk of being pre-term, your doctor or midwife may prescribe sexual abstinence after the second trimester. If this is an issue for either you or your partner, make sure you discuss it with each other and with your doctor.

ANOTHER MUM SAYS   'I think libido decreases in proportion to your stomach increasing. It depends on how you feel. Some of us feel great, most of us feel like crap.'

Choosing your medical team

Most people select their doctor, obstetrician or hospital based on referral or recommendation. Your choice of doctor might determine in which hospital your babies will be born, and whether you are a public or private patient. When you're meeting your doctor and/or midwife, make sure you ask them how many twin pregnancies they've looked after and how many twins they've brought into the world. Specialist care may be available from a doctor or obstetrician with multiple birth expertise. If you're not confident, don't hesitate to change your doctor. This pregnancy is different and specialist care may be beneficial. You could also ask about their treatment practices and birth preferences to see if those align with your own preferences.

Additional questions to ask your doctor or obstetrician might include:
- The fees charged for every aspect of your care and the care of your babies. If you have private health cover, find out how much you will be out of pocket.
- In which hospital will you give birth and why?
- Does this hospital have a Neonatal Intensive Care Unit (NICU) or Special Care Nursery? If not, where would you go if you have pre-term labour? Or where would your babies be sent if they are pre-term ?
- What symptoms might indicate pre-term labour?
- Are you likely to have a vaginal or caesarean birth? And why?
- What is likely to happen during labour and birth?
- Does your doctor use forceps or vacuum-assisted birth? What experience do they have in using these?
- What is the likelihood of your being given an episiotomy and when would that be decided?
- Will you be able to hold your babies immediately after their birth?
- What pain relief should you plan for?

The Royal Women's Hospital in Melbourne has a specialist multiple birth pregnancy clinic where they see both public and private health patients. Hospitals in other areas are planning to establish similar clinics. Multiple-birth clinics usually have many different medical and support staff, including midwives, dieticians, physiotherapists, obstetricians and paediatricians with a specific interest in multiple pregnancies and births, which can help parents to feel more confident and informed. Contact the main maternity hospital in your area for information on doctors and obstetricians with multiple pregnancy expertise.

You could find out if your hospital has a Neonatal Intensive Care Unit (NICU) and/or a Special Care Nursery. If your babies are pre-term they might need these facilities. If the hospital you plan to go to does not have these facilities, find out which ones do. If you go into labour early it may be best to get yourself to the hospital with special care for pre-term babies.

Investigate your chosen hospital's antenatal courses. These are usually free. Classes are for talking about and preparing for labour and birth. They teach you and your partner what to expect, ways to relax and how to give each other emotional support. You may like to enrol during your second trimester in case your babies arrive early. Many local branches of AMBA or NZMBA also offer antenatal sessions offering practical and emotional support and an opportunity to meet other expectant parents of multiples.

False alarms

If anything about your pregnancy is worrying you, even if you can't put your finger on it, call or visit your doctor or midwife. Do the same if you suspect you are going into labour. Don't worry about putting people out or feeling silly if it's a false alarm. It's important with a twin pregnancy to be extra cautious.

> (ANOTHER MUM SAYS)   'I had a scare five months into the pregnancy where I woke up one morning with a terrible pain, like a stitch, on my right side. After stretching and walking it wasn't going away. When I felt ill and threw up I rang the doctor, who said to come into emergency straightaway – he was on his way. I was dry-retching but as they started doing all the tests the pain suddenly disappeared and I felt a bit foolish. It was probably because of the weight of the babies that something got pinched while I slept on my side.'

Tests and procedures

Most women pregnant with twins will undergo regular tests and procedures. These tests help monitor the pregnancy, assess the health of your babies and pick up any problems that can be treated or prevented.

Urine tests

You may be asked to bring a urine sample with you or provide one at your regular appointments. Urine can be tested for protein regularly throughout your pregnancy. Protein in the urine can be a sign of kidney disease or of pre-eclampsia. Pre-eclampsia can be a serious pregnancy problem. See page 53 for more information. Urine can also be tested for ketones, which are by-products of fat breakdown. They can tell you whether your diet is lacking in carbohydrates or calories. Urine is also tested for sugar, which can be, but isn't always, an indicator for gestational diabetes. Most importantly, your urine is being checked for asymptomatic urinary tract infections.

Blood tests

Your blood can be checked for iron levels, Rh factor and infectious diseases. Your babies need adequate iron to form and grow properly. Carrying two babies drains more iron from your system so testing is carried out to discover if you have anaemia or low levels of iron in the blood. Your Rh factor is checked to thwart the potential for your body to make antibodies against your babies. You may also be tested for infectious diseases like HIV and Hepatitis B which cause potential problems for your babies if undiagnosed.

Pelvic examinations

This examination is done to determine the shape and angle of your cervix and uterus. In a healthy pregnancy this is often done on the first visit to a doctor or midwife. If you are experiencing any symptoms at other times a pelvic examination may be done.

Ultrasounds

Ultrasounds can be used to measure the due date, the growth of your babies and to check their internal and external organs. They can also be used to check on placental function and location, the sex of your babies, the volume of amniotic fluid and to check possible causes of vaginal bleeding. Sound waves show the babies, the placenta(s), the amniotic fluid and the membrane separating the babies (if there is one). The image is projected onto a video screen so that you can see it too.

Mothers of singletons usually have one or two ultrasounds during pregnancy whereas with a twin pregnancy you may have five or more.

ANOTHER MUM SAYS 'On one ultrasound I could see my little girl beating up her brother. She was using his head as a punching bag. It was hilarious.'

Foetal monitors

At check-ups your babies' heartbeats may be checked through a monitor placed on your tummy to make sure there are no signs of distress.

ANOTHER MUM SAYS 'I wanted a foetal monitor to take home so I could listen to my babies' heartbeats all day and all night. I was desperate to get to my doctors appointments to find out all was well.'

Tests for gestational diabetes

You are usually tested for gestational business between the 24th and 28th weeks of pregnancy using an oral glucose tolerance test. The test involves fasting overnight, having a high carbohydrate drink then later having your blood tested. If this result is abnormal the test is repeated in more detail.

If you have high levels of blood glucose you may be put on a special diet or be given insulin throughout your pregnancy. Gestational diabetes is at least twice as common in twin pregnancies as in single baby pregnancies.

Amniocentesis

During pregnancy, cells from the growing foetuses are shed into the amniotic fluid.

Amniocentesis involves inserting a needle, guided by ultrasound, through the pregnant belly and drawing out some amniotic fluid to evaluate the genetic material. The risk of miscarriage caused by amniocentesis is one in 200.

Many women expecting twins are in the 'older mother' category. Older mothers have an increased risk of genetic abnormalities so are often encouraged to have amniocentesis. Families with a history of chromosomal abnormalities are also encouraged to have amniocentesis testing.

Having the test is a personal decision for all couples. If chromosomal abnormalities are detected it may give you an opportunity to find out the implications of your family proceeding with the pregnancy. You will need straightforward information about your particular situation from medical advisers and counselling at the time and for as long as you feel it necessary.

ANOTHER MUM SAYS 'I'd done six IVF cycles to conceive these babies. Even though the risk of miscarriage was only one in 200 I wasn't going to take it. Regardless of the result I wouldn't terminate so there seemed no reason to have the test.'

ANOTHER MUM SAYS 'I had an amniocentesis because there was some concern my little girl had a thick neck, indicating abnormality. The test wasn't cheap. Medicare covers some of it but for twins we received a bill of over $1000. Nor was it a pleasant test. The needle hurts and I could feel it piercing the sac. I came home feeling ill and vomited, partly with worry. The results confirmed though that our little girl was OK so it was all worth the peace of mind.'

Chorionic villus sampling (CVS)

CVS testing serves the same purpose as amniocentesis, but can be done earlier in the pregnancy. CVS is often used to test for fragile X, a genetic disorder causing intellectual disability. Women who carry the fragile X gene are more likely to have twins. The procedure is very similar; congenital conditions can be tested for by sampling the chorionic villi, which are projections from the chorionic membrane and eventually form part of the placenta. They contain parts of your babies' genetic material. The risk of miscarriage caused by CVS testing is one in 100.

ANOTHER MUM SAYS 'The ultrasound doctor suggested an immediate CVS for both babies and within 15 minutes of arriving for a routine scan we had two lots of needles into my belly, meaning an increased risk of miscarriage. I left there very shaken and wondering why my life couldn't be more simple! The next 24 hours were hell. What would we do if one was abnormal or both? Would I again miscarry – this time with two babies? I didn't sleep a wink. I cried, I panicked and I secretly became excited about the possibility of two healthy wonderful babies. In my husband's style of 'being positive' he was sure it would all be OK. I sat by the phone all day and waited. The obstetrician said he'd call as soon as he had an initial result. The full result would take two weeks. It was the longest day of my life. By the time the call came my whole energy was focused on this outcome. Ethical dilemmas about what to do if one or both had chromosomal abnormalities had flashed through my mind. I had decided that if both babies had Down's syndrome we would terminate. How could we manage two special needs babies? How could we cope? As it happened the tests were completely clear. The apparent thickening of the neck (sometimes a sign of problems) was more a result of timing and position of the babies. I screamed with delight when the doctor pronounced our wonderful result.'

Cervical surveillance

If you have a history of giving birth prematurely or have had surgery to the cervix in the past, your doctor may advise 'cervical surveillance'. This can involve measuring the length of the cervix by vaginal ultrasound every week during the second trimester using a test called foetal fibronectin. This, combined with taking swabs from the vagina to test for any sign of infection which could precipitate premature labour, can help determine the likelihood of premature labour developing.

Pelvic floor muscle exercises

Exercise that vagina! You won't regret doing your pelvic floor exercises both during and after your pregnancy. Twins place an additional strain on your pelvic and abdominal muscles. Good strength 'down there' will make your life a lot easier – doing the exercises may prevent leaking when you laugh, cough and sneeze and will help get you back in shape after the birth. If you aren't already familiar with your pelvic floor muscles, stop the flow in the mid-stream of a pee – that's them! Tightening these muscles regularly will strengthen your pelvic floor. Once you are well-practised at pelvic floor exercises, you can do them every time you stop at the traffic lights, when you're on the phone or whenever you think about George Clooney.

Perineal massage

The perineum (the area between the anus and the vagina) stretches during a vaginal birth. Massaging this area daily from 34–36 weeks may make the area more supple and can decrease the chance of tearing or possibly the need for an episiotomy.

Exercising everything else

You will need a lot of fitness and stamina for the birth and caring for your babies. Discuss with your medical advisers the state of your health for exercise and any restrictions you should consider. There are specific exercise groups for pregnant women run by physiotherapists and fitness leaders trained in pregnancy. They can guide you depending on your special needs and energy levels. Some hospitals offer special antenatal and postnatal exercise classes where you're guided through appropriate stretch and relaxation exercises.

After your second trimester, you may be encouraged to rest as much as possible. If you are used to having a solid and regular exercise regime you may need to slow down and avoid overheating. Make sure you discuss an exercise plan with your medical adviser.

Rest

During the first few weeks of a twin pregnancy you may only have the energy to work and sleep. You may not even be able do that much. It's the body adjusting to its pregnant state and the changing levels of hormones. You may have more energy in the second trimester (weeks 13–24) but again from week 25 you'll probably start to feel tired. Twin pregnancies can be the size of a full term single pregnancy by the sixth or seventh month. You'll probably need more rest as time passes. Rest is also very important in determining the size of your babies. Some experts recommend resting for six hours a day when you reach 28 weeks, as well as resting overnight.

Consider giving yourself a regular early bedtime and try not to let anything disrupt it. Put the answering machine on, grab your hotty, your chamomile tea and your trashy novel and roll into bed.

If you have older children, call in favours from friends with children and/or consider using childcare, even if it's just one day a week

If you're employed outside the home:
- Cut back your hours at work.
- Email everything, even to the person in the next room.
- Ask anyone walking past to get things for you.
- Have a stool under your desk to put your feet up.
- Organise someone else to do all lifting and heavy work.
- Ask for regular hours on shift work so your body isn't constantly readjusting.
- If you have no pregnancy complications, consider leaving work. before 28 weeks and resting for six hours a day after that.

REST TIPS

- Lie down at the first hint of dizziness and at any other time you can – blood flow to you and your babies is better when you're horizontal.
- Sit down and put your feet up when you can.
- Put daytime naps in your daily schedule, and if you have older children, rest when they do.
- Have fruit and vegies, groceries, chemist things, and anything else you can think of, delivered.
- Buy healthy takeaway food.
- Prioritise your social engagements and commitments and ditch all unnecessary activities.

Relaxation

Yoga, meditation or visualisation can be a great way to relax during a twin pregnancy. There are many different forms of yoga, some more appropriate during pregnancy than others, so check first with your instructor.

15 MINUTE RELAXATION TIP:

- Lie down in a dark and quiet room with blankets an eye bag, some oils burning and the phone off the hook.
- Breath slowly in and out of your nose.
- Focus on your breath going in and out of your body.
- Feel your breath inflating and deflating your lungs.
- Imagine your breath sustaining your cells.
- Begin to relax your muscles by tensing them on the in breath and relaxing them on your out breath. Start with the muscles in your toes, working up your ankles, shins, thighs etc.
- If you're still awake by the time you reach your forehead, then enjoy your peaceful state

Easing discomforts and dealing with difficulties

Building two babies and carrying a double load is a lot of work. Hormonal changes occurring during pregnancy can increase your vulnerability to injury. Advice from physiotherapists, especially those dealing in women's health, can be very beneficial during pregnancy. Often symptoms for different problems can present similarly so careful assessment is needed.

Aches and pains are normal but any lingering pain needs individual assessment and treatment.

Can't sleep a wink?

Many pregnant women have trouble sleeping and those expecting two babies can have even more difficulty, especially in the third trimester. You may be absolutely exhausted but still not be able to nod off, maybe because of muscle aches and pains, perhaps due to the babies moving or pressure on the bladder causing you to get up a lot to go to the loo. Or you may be thinking and worrying. Sleeping on your side (the side of you, not the bed) is important, as the weight of the babies squashes the large blood vessels in your abdomen if you sleep on your back and can cause a drop in blood pressure when you stand up. If you find you've rolled onto your back in your sleep don't panic – your body will compensate and you'll roll back onto your side.

It doesn't matter when you sleep, only that you do. If you can't sleep at night, try to arrange to sleep in the day. Let your body guide you.

TO HELP YOU NOD OFF

- Have a snack and drink chamomile tea or warm milk before bed.
- Have a warm shower.
- Have a bedtime routine – go to bed at the same time each night.
- Sleep in really clean sheets.
- Sprinkle diluted lavender oil on the pillow.
- An egg crate style foam pad on top of your mattress can distribute your weight more evenly.
- Have lots of pillows, or a body pillow, handy to put under your knees, hips or tummy to help you get comfortable. Pillows between the legs can help a lot.
- If you must sleep on your back sit up a bit with a pile of pillows.
- Keep a pen and paper handy so you can remind yourself what to worry about in the morning.

ANOTHER MUM SAYS 'Being awake all night really upset me. It would build up and build up, then I'd cry and it was like a release, finally I'd go to sleep. Towards the end I felt I didn't need to keep day/night cycles. Once I surrendered to it and accepted that I would be awake all night, I stopped getting upset.'

Body temperature

During pregnancy your metabolism works faster and your body temperature often rises. To keep comfortable, dress appropriately – even if you're wearing a T-shirt while everyone else is in jumpers; shower often or wash your hands and feet to help keep yourself cool.

Morning sickness and nausea

Morning sickness is not completely understood but one possible cause is the placenta producing the hormone HCG, while falling blood pressure is another. In a twin pregnancy these changes are greater, so morning sickness can be more extreme. About a third of mothers with single baby pregnancies experience morning sickness compared to half or more of mothers expecting twins. The good news is it usually only lasts for the first trimester.

It is called morning sickness because many women are sick in the morning but it can happen at any time of day. It can be just a queasy feeling, incapacitating vomiting or anything in between. Not feeling hungry is also a form of nausea.

Extreme morning sickness is called hyperemesis gravidarum and can cause liver and kidney damage. You'll know if you have it, you'll be unable to keep anything down and you'll lose weight. The immediate danger is dehydration. Your doctor may prescribe anti-nausea medication. In more extreme cases, you could be hospitalised and have an IV drip to replace lost fluids and prevent dehydration.

TO TREAT NAUSEA AND VOMITING

- Get plenty of rest and sleep.
- Graze all day.
- Try eating dry toast or biscuits when you wake up but before you sit up.
- Eat high carbohydrate food – bread, potatoes, pasta, noodles and rice.
- Drink plenty of fluids, especially water, drinking between rather than with meals.
- Have a snack before bed and/or at 2 a.m.
- Keep a diary of what makes you feel ill to figure out what you can eat.
- Stay away from smells that make you queasy, get someone else to cook.
- Fatty foods can make it much worse.
- Try acupressure, B6 tablets, barley sugar, ginger tablets or ginger tea.

ANOTHER MUM SAYS   'By week eight I couldn't even keep water down and lost six kilos in one week. I was admitted to hospital and after 24 hours on the drip I began to recover. My middle trimester was great but I started vomiting again in my last month, which really hurt.'

Indigestion and heartburn

Your babies are squashing your insides and your pregnancy hormones are slowing down your digestion. It's no wonder so many women carrying twins have indigestion in the third trimester. If your heartburn is severe, discuss it with your doctor as you may need medication.

TO RELIEVE THAT PAINFUL BURNING

- Drink icy cold milk.
- Try peppermint tea.
- Graze all day.
- If you can stomach it, Swedish Bitters is available from the health food store.
- A famous Greek remedy is eating sesame seeds.
- Fried and fatty foods make it worse.
- Elevate the head of your bed.
- If it's too much to bear try over-the-counter medicines but check with your doctor first to find out which ones are OK.

Haemorrhoids and constipation

If you are straining when you go to the toilet then you are constipated. It's not how often, it's how difficult. Constipation occurs when progesterone relaxes your muscles and causes your digestion to slow down. The food in your system takes longer on its journey and dries out along the way.

Don't be embarrassed when the veins in your bottom start popping out because of the pressure of your babies. Haemorrhoids happen more often and more severely in twin pregnancies. They are varicose veins of the anal canal and you'll know you've got them when you can feel little lumps around your anus. Pelvic floor muscle exercises can help with haemorrhoids. See page 38. If there are traces of blood, you should see the doctor, as the anus can split and be difficult to heal. A prescribed cortisone cream usually solves the splitting problem. Avoiding constipation is a huge help with haemorrhoids.

TIPS FOR AVOIDING AND TREATING HAEMORRHOIDS

- Drink at least two litres of water per day and avoid coffee.
- See a physiotherapist who specialises in women's health.
- Eat plenty of fruit and vegies.
- Eat food with lots of fibre like bread, rice, grains and cereal.
- Eat spicy foods and chilies.
- Get some exercise.
- Use ice packs on haemorrhoids on your bottom.

If this doesn't work, you may need pharmacy or prescription medicines and ointments, but check first with your medical adviser

Varicose veins in your legs

Varicose veins are unnaturally and permanently distended veins. They are magnified in twin pregnancies. Keep your feet up as much as possible and put support stockings on before you get up to improve varicose veins in the legs.

Vulval varicose veins

Pelvic floor muscle exercises (see page 38) done early in pregnancy may help varicosity. There's no way of avoiding vulval varicose veins, and they are more likely to occur in a twin pregnancy. A pressure garment is available from physios – specially designed undies that support varicosity.

Round ligament pain

The round ligaments hold your uterus inside your hips. As your babies grow, these ligaments have to stretch a lot, and this can cause spasms.

The hormones loosening up your pelvis to prepare it for labour can also loosen the ligaments around your other joints, including hips, knees and those in the feet. They can present as a dull ache or the spasms as they stretch can be felt as shooting pains.

REDUCING ROUND LIGAMENT PAIN

- Wear flat, comfortable, bouncy shoes.
- Move gently and try not to twist.
- Have warm baths.
- Lie down with pillows supporting the weight of your tummy.
- Hold a pillow round your tummy then roll out of bed, like a log.

Pelvic joint pain

Pelvic joint pain is hormonal in its basis.

> **ANOTHER MUM SAYS** 'Pelvic joint pain made my pubic bone feel like it was bruised. It started with back pain and they said it might come around to the front, which it did. I was doing yoga thinking it would make it better but it was making it worse. I avoided walking up hills and up stairs, avoided separating my legs, had massages and hot baths, and took paracetamol sometimes.

Instability of the pelvis

During pregnancy hormones that are working to soften or relax your supportive ligaments and muscles can make your pelvis unstable. Don't take the stairs – this can make the pelvis more unstable and painful, if you must take the stairs walk up them sideways. Seek advice from a women's health physio on how to move and how to use a support belt.

Back ache

The size of your belly means your back is taking a lot of extra weight. Muscles keep your bones in position so if you strengthen your muscles you may save your back. Good back muscle strengthening exercises include swimming, yoga or the Alexander Technique. Your back will be under enormous strain while lifting, changing and caring for your babies. Consider seeing a physiotherapist for advice before any problems occur. You may only need a single visit.

If you have back pain – and many women expecting twins do – don't take any medication without speaking with your doctor first. Contractions can begin as persistent backache. If you feel your backache is persistent or different than usual, consult your doctor or midwife.

> **ANOTHER MUM SAYS** 'My osteopath became my best friend during my twin pregnancy. He gently adjusted my hips and lower back, checked my spine was OK and that there wasn't tension in my neck. The most amazing thing he did was to gently manipulate my organs allowing my diaphragm room to expand so I could breathe easier.'

CARING FOR YOUR BACK

- Wear low heeled shoes.
- When standing, don't let your back sway forward. Tuck your hips under and let your pelvis and legs support your weight.
- Stand for two hours maximum during early pregnancy and an hour at a time later.
- Keep your back straight and elevate your legs when sitting in a chair.
- Alternate putting one foot up on a small stool or step when possible.
- Use a fit ball to sit as this helps strengthen your back. It's very important to make sure it's the correct size.
- When lifting, bend your knees and keep your back straight.
- Sitting on a stool under a hot shower or a warm bath can relax your muscles and soothe any pain, heat packs applied to the painful area can help, or have a massage or ask your partner to rub your back.
- If you have large breasts, a good well-fitted bra can ease the strain on your back.
- Choose cots, highchairs, prams and equipment carefully so that they are at the right height for you.
- You can get 'maternity supports' from physiotherapists which might be appropriate, depending on the assessment of your symptoms.
- Relaxation and gentle exercise help stiffness and backache.
- Some yoga exercises can relieve backache. Get down on your hands and knees, push your back up high and stretch, then push your belly towards the floor.
- Make sure you tell your doctor or midwife about any back pain.

Leg and foot cramps

Leg and foot cramps in pregnancy are caused by increased pressure from your belly on your leg nerves. They happen at night and can often wake you suddenly from a deep sleep. The first one can give you quite a shock. If there is someone in bed with you, get them to gently push your toes towards your shin, then rub your leg or foot to relieve the cramp. If you're alone, you'll have to get into a position where you can gently pull it out yourself. Sometimes the cramp will go, then as soon as you relax it comes back. Massage and leg and foot stretching exercises can help to avoid cramps.

Restless legs and leaping feet

Some pregnant women's legs seem to jump around all night, making it impossible for them to get much sleep. The more physically tired you are, the more your legs leap. Your natural urge is to try to stop them leaping but resisting the movements makes them worse so it can be better to let them jump.

TIPS FOR RELIEVING THE LEAPS

- Have a warm shower or bath when your legs are restless.
- Have a massage – some hospitals have cheap or free massages for their patients.
- Avoid chocolate, coffee, tea, alcohol and soft drinks.
- Try to get plenty of sleep so you're not overtired.
- Paracetamol may give temporary relief.

Oedema (swollen hands and feet)

Most pregnant women have swollen fingers, hands, ankles and/or feet because pregnancy increases the volume of blood. Legs can also swell due to the heavy uterus placing pressure on the major vein which is returning blood to your heart for oxygenation. This means the blood flow to the legs slows down, resulting in oedema. Progesterone is also a factor as it causes veins and muscles to relax, similarly resulting in blood taking longer to return to the heart.

The swelling can put pressure on nerves in the wrists causing carpal tunnel syndrome. There's pain, numbness and tingling in the thumb and fingers. It can be in one or both hands and usually goes away after the birth. A splint on the wrist usually relieves the pain.

If this swelling is sudden or severe or not just around the hands and feet contact your doctor or midwife, as it may be a sign of pre-eclampsia and could become serious. See Possible complications, page 49.

TIPS FOR RELIEVING THE SWELLING

- Drink lots of water.
- Lie on your side.
- Put your feet up as often as possible.
- Soak your feet in a bath or a foot spa then rub peppermint lotion into your feet.

- Try dandelion *leaf* tea – it must be leaf, not plain dandelion tea or dandelion root tea (which are not recommended in pregnancy).
- Wear comfy or no shoes and don't wear socks or stockings that cut off circulation.
- Take your rings off and put them somewhere safe.
- Don't reduce your salt intake. If you do, your kidneys will try to retain salt and will retain more water with it.

Shortness of breath

The bigger you get, the less room your lungs have to expand for breathing. You're also carrying extra weight and extra fluid. You can get puffed out walking to the mail box, talking, or even when you're resting on the couch. You need more oxygen when you're pregnant so your breathing rate increases even when you're sleeping.

IF YOU ARE BREATHLESS

- Go slow.
- Stop and rest.
- Sit and stand up straight.
- Avoid activities that leave you short of breath.
- If breathing is difficult when you're lying down, prop lots of pillows under your head and shoulders.
- If you are having chest pains or are finding it hard to breathe, contact your doctor, as this may be a sign of something more serious.

Skin things

Stretchmarks can be pink, red, purple or pale brown and itch like mad and they're often hereditary. There's not much you can do to avoid them. They're a common occurrence in the very stretched tummy skin of a twin pregnancy. They can appear on your breasts, tummy, hips, thighs and bottom. They turn silver and are barely noticeable after a few years.

Other skin changes that occur in pregnancy are skin pigmentation, especially on the face, new moles, darker nipples, oilier skin, skin tags, broken blood vessels and a dark line called linea nigra heading down from your belly button.

> ### TIPS FOR RELIEVING ITCHY TUMMIES AND SKIN CHANGES
>
> - Using sunscreen on your face reduces the appearance of chloasma (skin pigmentation on the face).
> - Creams keep your skin moist and lessen the itch but there's no guarantee they'll reduce the number or severity of stretch-marks.
> - Glycerine rubbed on your tummy overnight means you'll wake up with wonderful soft belly skin.
> - Wearing cotton clothes can ease the itching.
> - Oatmeal baths may relieve the itch. They are made by popping a stocking of oatmeal under the running water in your bath.
> - Rubbing lavender oil or petroleum jelly on your belly can also lessen the itch.
> - Using non-soap products instead of soap may also help.
>
> *If the itch is severe, please talk to your doctor.*

Possible complications

Most of the following complications are more common in a twin pregnancy than in a single baby pregnancy. There's no reason to think that they will happen to you but it's sensible to be aware of the possible symptoms. Recognising the warning signs gives you an opportunity to contact your medical adviser. Some complications can be dangerous if left untreated, while early treatment often leads to a better outcome.

Small-for-dates babies

'Small-for-dates' is another term for 'intrauterine growth restriction' (IUGR). This means one or both of your babies is smaller than average. For some reason, twins born at a lower birth weight have less health problems than single babies born at a lower birth weight. One third of all twins are small-for-dates. Sometimes one twin is significantly smaller than the other.

IUGR is diagnosed through ultrasound measurements of babies. It can be caused by a poor diet or low weight-gain in the mother, or it can indicate that there are problems with the placenta, or that the babies have 'twin-to-twin transfusion' syndrome (see page 58). Or there may be none of these problems present, it may just be genetic.

If one or both of your babies are small-for-dates, you may be put on bed rest, be given a high calorie diet and the babies, their placentas and amniotic sacs will probably be monitored very closely. Your doctor will know if your twins are growing adequately. An early birth is sometimes necessary.

Pre-term labour

Pre-term labour and birth is the most common complication of a twin pregnancy. For twins between 35 and 38 weeks is considered the optimum length for the pregnancy, with the average twin pregnancy lasting 36 weeks.

Pre-term labour means your babies are trying to come early. Depending on how early, your doctors may want to try to stop the labour. It's really important to get treatment as soon as possible – the birth may be able to be delayed using drugs to stop your contractions. This may give your babies a chance to stay inside for a bit longer and an easier start to life. If you are given Nifedipine or any other drug to stop labour, you will probably be admitted to hospital so that both you and your babies can be monitored closely. It is usually given by injection but when labour is being stopped over a long time it can be in oral form.

RECOGNISING THE SIGNS OF EARLY LABOUR

- Five or more contractions in an hour.
- Rhythmic or persistent pressure on the pelvis.
- A feeling like period cramps.
- Lower back pain that persists or begins suddenly.
- A change in the colour amount or consistency of vaginal discharge.
- Your waters breaking – it may be a slow leak or a gush, the wetness smells sweet, is pale and straw coloured and continues to leak. When you stand up one baby's head may cork the leak but when you lie down or move it'll start leaking again.
- Diarrhoea can be a sign of labour, so call your doctor.
- A 'bloody show' when the plug comes out of the cervix and you have a pink mucus discharge. It may mean labour is about to start or it could mean labour is weeks away.
- A feeling that something isn't right is always worth checking out. A lot of women say this was their only warning sign.

If you have any one of these signs contact your medical adviser immediately.

Steroids are also often given by injection if pre-term labour is being delayed. Two doses are given 12–24 hours apart. The steroids help the babies' lungs mature before birth, provided labour can be stopped at least for that 48 hours. The steroids form a layer of fat and protein on the inside of the babies' lungs so they can breathe more easily once out in the air.

Anaemia

Iron deficiency anaemia means a lack of iron in your blood. Iron allows red blood cells to carry oxygen around our bodies. Your pregnant body produces a much greater volume of blood but doesn't increase its level of iron. This extra blood dilutes the amount of oxygen travelling around your body, making you feel more tired and sluggish. A lack of iron can contribute to pre-term births and low birth weights.

Check with your medical adviser before taking an iron supplement. Natural and organic iron supplements are available from health food stores and are less likely to cause constipation. Slow-release iron supplements are also less likely to cause constipation and nausea. If you are prescribed an iron supplement, taking it with vitamin C gives maximum absorption. Taking it with a meal stops it irritating your stomach. Don't take your iron with tea, coffee or caffeine drinks, as this will reduce the level of absorption.

Gestational diabetes

Gestational diabetes is diabetes that usually occurs in the second half of pregnancy. Pregnancy causes an increase in blood-sugar levels and a twin pregnancy increases these levels even more. Sometimes the body doesn't produce enough insulin to regulate these higher blood-sugar levels, causing gestational diabetes. The placenta can also produce hormones that cause your body to resist the insulin.

Women with a family history of diabetes are more prone to gestational diabetes. It is usually discovered through a glucose tolerance test.

Symptoms of gestational diabetes include excessive thirst, frequent urinating, an increased volume of wee and feeling very tired. Treatment involves monitoring your diet and strictly controlling calorie and carbohydrate intake. This usually controls the glucose levels. You may be given a low dose of self-administered insulin injections. The diabetes is usually temporary and disappears after you give birth, but your babies need to be monitored closely for respiratory problems and hypoglycaemia. If you have had gestational diabetes, you should watch your post-pregnancy diet as you are more at risk of developing non-gestational diabetes.

> ANOTHER MUM SAYS   'The news that I had gestational diabetes came as an absolute shock to me. I became really angry and quite emotional. Prior to both my twin pregnancy and previous single pregnancy I had begun eating really well. I avoided caffeine, alcohol and highly processed foods containing lots of sugar, salt and fats. I'm always healthiest when I'm pregnant and suddenly I was being told that I had gestational diabetes and that my diet had to be looked at and modified. Now more than ever I really had to eat good food and avoid the hidden sugars as much as possible. I also had to do the dreaded reading of my blood-sugar levels three times a day for the rest of my pregnancy. The test had to be done half an hour after every meal no matter where I was. My consultant checked the results like homework at every visit. My blood-sugar levels were apparently excellent for a pregnant woman with gestational diabetes. One day I complained to my doctor about my Claytons condition and I was moaning about doing the blood-sugar tests. She quickly put me in my place by reminding me that I was genuinely diagnosed, however mildly, with the condition, and with a multiple pregnancy nothing can be ignored or left to chance.'

If you have diabetes prior to your twin pregnancy, and it's not controlled, it can affect the babies. They can put on too much weight and are more susceptible to hypoglycaemia and respiratory distress syndrome at birth. Birth defects and stillbirth are more common in cases of uncontrolled diabetes, but are still very rare for twins because twin pregnancies are monitored very closely, especially where diabetes is present.

Chronic itching
The belly of a twin pregnancy stretches and itches. There are two causes of chronic itching: PUPPP (pruritic urticarial papules and plaques of pregnancy) and obstetric cholestasis. See your doctor immediately if you suspect either of these. PUPPP begins looking like stretch-marks and may be caused by a suddenly stretched tummy.

It quickly becomes bumpy with scaly patches and is unbearably itchy. Doctors often prescribe antihistamines or steroids for relief.

Obstetric cholestasis is a potentially serious complication of pregnancy and is more common in twin pregnancies. It usually occurs during the third trimester and presents as itching all over without a rash. The itching is often worse at night. It usually develops on the soles of the feet and the palms of the hands then spreads to the trunk and limbs. The exact cause is unknown but one theory is that it's caused by the liver ducts slowing or becoming blocked in pregnancy and not processing the bile salts in the body. Cholestasis causes an increased risk of pre-term delivery, foetal distress and in less than two per cent of cases, stillbirth.

Cholestasis can also cause disruption to the absorption of fat-soluble vitamins, especially vitamin K which is needed for clotting to avoid a haemorrhage after your babies are born. Close monitoring, drug treatment and planned early delivery are the most common treatments. The symptoms usually disappear soon after birth.

Pre-eclampsia

Pre-eclampsia is a condition related to pregnancy where your blood pressure rises suddenly, your hands, face and feet swell from retained fluid and protein appears in your urine. Be aware of the warning signs of pre-eclampsia as severe cases can cause the babies' blood supply to be inadequate so they don't receive enough nutrients.

Pre-eclampsia occurs in 15 per cent of twin pregnancies. The risk is higher if this is your first pregnancy, if you are an 'older' mother, if you had high blood pressure before the pregnancy or if you have diabetes, kidney disease or are not eating well. Let your doctor know if you have had high blood pressure in the past or if members of your family have, or have had, high blood pressure.

Pre-eclampsia is more common in the second half of pregnancy and usually disappears not long after the babies are born. In some cases it doesn't develop until during or after delivery.

If pre-eclampsia is diagnosed, the treatment depends on how severe it is. It may be observation, bed rest, maybe some hospital rest, a low salt diet, medication or possibly labour being induced or a caesarean.

If untreated pre-eclampsia can lead to eclampsia in the mother, a very dangerous condition for mother and babies, so it's important to be aware of all the possible signs.

CONTACT YOUR DOCTOR IMMEDIATELY IF ANY OF THE FOLLOWING WARNING SIGNS APPEAR

- More than minor swelling in your hands, feet and face
- Sudden swelling in your hands, feet and face
- Sudden weight gain
- Severe headaches and dizziness
- Blurry vision or seeing spots
- Nausea or vomiting
- Stomach pains
- Pain under your breastbone or right side
- Infrequent or inability to pee

ANOTHER MUM SAYS   'My blood pressure was always being monitored and seemed an issue with my doctor. At around three to four months pre-eclampsia was finally diagnosed following a 24-hour urine test. I was given two huge bottles to fill up over the following day. I couldn't go to work or do anything but stay at home pouring it down one end and collecting it at the other. When the test results came back I was put on medication. I never felt sick and didn't know I had high blood pressure. It was quite funny that throughout my pregnancy my babies passed all their tests with flying colours – growing at the right rate, heads down, doing really well – while as the mother, I was failing each test.

Part of the reason I was induced at 37 weeks was because my blood pressure had risen again. It was carefully monitored during the birth and immediately afterwards. The problem completely disappeared about a day later.'

Enforced bed rest

Some women are told by their medical adviser to put their feet up for days, weeks or months. If this happens you may feel guilty, scared, dependent, bored, isolated, lonely, depressed or relieved. People who live in the country and are admitted to hospital for weeks prior to the birth are in a particularly difficult and disruptive situation for their entire family.

Many women on bed rest find it helpful to have a routine to their day.

Here are some ideas to help you through this temporary period.

- Have a phone, snacks and water by the bed.
- Keep your pyjamas on – people expect nothing from you and offer more help when you're wearing PJs.
- Read the entire paper every day, read lots of trashy novels and watch TV.
- Take up cryptic crosswords.
- Sort photos into albums and recipes into books.
- Write letters and keep a diary.
- Get a lap top and start emailing.
- Order the next 12 months worth of Christmas and birthday presents online.
- Update your address book then address birthday, Christmas, Hannukkah and thank you cards.
- Organise friends and family so they don't all visit at once.
- Arrange friends to come and visit for a bedside chat. If you're allowed to be driven around, lie on a friend's couch.
- Organise a mobile massage, facial, manicure or haircut.
- Just be quiet and listen to your body.

ANOTHER MUM SAYS   'I wasn't sick but my condition was serious enough to warrant me staying in hospital. I would have been induced the moment things worsened. Sadly, this was the only time I felt truly pampered during my pregnancy. I rested and really began to focus on the impending arrival of our twins. This was such a precious time to prepare myself mentally and physically for all that was about to begin. I spent a lot of time in the nursery with the beautiful newborns and talking to all the mums and nurses. By the time the day arrived to have my twin daughters I was truly prepared. I felt focused, rested and excited. While nobody wants complications during pregnancy my hypertension was the catalyst for some positive things. I know I wouldn't have been half as rested or psyched if I'd spent the last weeks of my pregnancy charging around the house and town trying to keep up with everything and everybody. As a wife and mother it's very hard to put yourself first and to listen to the needs of your body. Staying in hospital forced me to slow down and truly relish those final weeks of pregnancy.'

(ANOTHER MUM SAYS)   'I stayed in hospital to rest and was closely watched for any developments. Because I was nearing the end of my pregnancy I was grateful for this time-out away from the demands of a busy household and energetic toddler. I was simply not getting the rest I needed at home. My doctor knew this and I felt as though she was doing me a favour. She also 'ordered' little escapes to get fresh air and sunshine – such as coffee with friends and a couple of family picnics.'

Premature rupturing of membranes or 'waters breaking'

If water leaks or gushes from your vagina or if you feel a constant wetness in your pants, your membranes may have broken and you may be going into labour. Contact your hospital, doctor or midwife. Waters breaking before 37 weeks is considered premature rupturing of membranes.

Once your waters have broken your babies are susceptible to infection. It may be dangerous for you and the babies to wait, so don't hesitate. If you're going to hospital, put a maternity pad in your pants and take a towel or two with you for the journey.

You will most likely be given antibiotics to prevent infection, and steroids over two days to help mature your babies' lungs. If your membranes rupture very early in the pregnancy, the birth will be delayed for as long as possible.

Vaginal bleeding

The cervix has an increased blood supply in pregnancy and can readily bleed. If there is not much blood and no pain, it may be post-coital bleeding Any signs of bleeding should be checked with your medical adviser.

Bleeding in the first trimester: In early pregnancy bleeding associated with or followed by cramping, period-type pain or backache may indicate threatened or complete miscarriage. It's always best to consult your doctor if you have any bleeding.

In the second trimester: Light bleeding usually doesn't indicate big problems in the second and third trimesters but always contact your doctor or midwife. Bleeding sometimes indicates an 'incompetent cervix', when the cervix opens spontaneously, and this can result in late miscarriage. Treatment involves putting a stitch (suture) in the cervix, and sometimes bed rest, until it's time to give birth.

Later bleeding: In late pregnancy, pain and heavy bleeding can be a sign of placenta praevia or placental abruption (see below). Abruption is usually always associated with pain, which could be in addition to bleeding or without any bleeding at all.

Placenta praevia

This is the term used to describe when the placenta is very low in the uterus and covering part of the cervix. This can happen in a single pregnancy but is more common with twins as there is more placenta in the uterus. It is usually diagnosed during an ultrasound. Placenta praevia that is disturbed by moving babies can cause painless bleeding. If that happens it's usually late in the pregnancy when the uterus is stretching and your cervix is preparing for the birth.

Bed rest is usually prescribed, sometimes in hospital. If you lose a large amount of blood you may need a blood transfusion and a caesarean section. Always tell your doctor or midwife if you bleed even if you feel no pain.

Placental abruption

This occurs when the placenta separates from the wall of the uterus before the birth of your babies. A twin pregnancy is about three times more likely to have placental abruption than a singleton. This may sound like a lot but it isn't very common. Placental abruption causes medium to heavy vaginal bleeding and medium to severe pain. High blood pressure, smoking and not eating properly increase your risk of the placenta separating early.

If the placenta completely separates it is very dangerous as the babies' supply of oxygen and nourishment is cut off. Contractions can begin when abruption occurs, and the pain and bleeding will tell you that something's not right. Sometimes a concealed abruption will be painful without the vaginal bleeding. Go to hospital immediately or contact your doctor.

Amniotic fluid problems

The babies float in, swallow and pee out amniotic fluid. These are the 'waters' that eventually break. The amount of fluid in each amniotic sac is measured at your ultrasound appointments and too much or too little indicates a problem. If you have these amniotic fluid problems you will be monitored very closely until the birth.

Too much fluid in the amniotic sac (polyhydramnios) is common in cases of twin-to-twin transfusion (see below). The extra fluid in the uterus can cause waters to break early and pre-term labour. Amniocentesis is often used to remove excess fluid.

Too little fluid in the amniotic sac (oligohydramnios) is more common when there is one placenta and twin-to-twin transfusion. Low amniotic fluid levels can also mean small-for-dates babies. We can't add fluid to the amniotic sac but if the problem is twin-to-twin transfusion, removing fluid from the sac with too much can help stimulate the one without enough to produce more fluid.

Twin to twin transfusion syndrome

This condition can only happen in the 65 per cent of MZ twin pregnancies where the babies share a placenta. Twin-to-twin transfusion tends to happen in 15 per cent of these twins.

When there is twin-to-twin transfusion syndrome, the blood in the placenta is only flowing one way. It flows from one baby through the umbilical cord to the cord of the other baby, but not back. This means one baby receives more nutrition. The baby going without is also losing blood and can develop anaemia, become 'small-for-dates' and have too little fluid in the amniotic sac. The baby receiving more nutrition receives too much blood, grows too big, can develop heart failure, organ failure and too much fluid in the amniotic sac. The earlier this transfusion occurs the more dangerous it is so twin-to-twin transfusion needs to be treated as soon as it is detected. If your babies have one placenta and one outer membrane surrounding them, the placenta will probably be monitored constantly via ultrasound.

The nuchal translucency test which measures the thickness of the skin on the back of the baby's neck can be a very useful predicator of twin to twin transfusion. This test has traditionally been done as a screening test to detect Down syndrome at around twelve weeks gestation.

If you and your babies are being treated for twin-to-twin transfusion, you may have amniocentesis to remove extra amniotic fluid from the bigger baby. This can also make you more physically comfortable and reduce the risk of pre-term labour. It may need to be done regularly throughout your pregnancy.

Another treatment for twin-to-twin transfusion is laser surgery on the placenta, sealing shut the connecting blood vessels between the umbilical cords. This is only done in severe cases between 18 and 26 weeks. If the problem is not improving, giving birth to your babies early may be the only option.

ANOTHER MUM SAYS   'Having twins for the first time, I thought everything that seemed abnormal was just because it was twins. At my appointment at 25 weeks, my doctor said that he wanted me to go and have a scan immediately as he was worried about my fluid levels. The technician was panicking and said I was going to have to go into hospital. I was wondering how my family was going to manage with me in hospital for 12 weeks. I was also so sore and sick that I really didn't know how I was going to get through it.

I had no idea my babies were about to be born. I was told that the larger of the babies was in real trouble. There was too much amniotic fluid and his heart could not cope with pumping it around. We were advised that the smaller twin would have a better chance and that he'd be tougher and stronger. We were presented with three options. Firstly, do nothing, in which case both babies would probably die soon. Secondly, wait 24 hours take steroids and probably lose the bigger baby in utero, while the smaller would have some chance. Thirdly, have a caesarean tonight and try to save both babies. I didn't really feel like there was any option but to try to save both babies. We were advised that the hospital had two beds in NICU. I just thought 'of course' without realising then how lucky we were to get two NICU places in the same hospital. Some babies are sent interstate in these situations. When I came out of the general, the first thing the doctor said to me was, 'We've got two live babies.' I felt that meant we were off to a good start. After my boys were born one of the first things I wanted to know was whether I'd be able to have more children. I wanted to be able to get it right next time. I've heard other mothers of premmies say the same thing.'

Umbilical cord problems

When identical twins share an amniotic sac there is a chance that the umbilical cords will become tangled. It is a dangerous complication and can result in death of one or both babies. If you have two babies in one amniotic sac, you should be monitored closely throughout your pregnancy. An early caesarean may be needed if the cords become tangled. Make sure you trust your doctor or midwife and feel you are being watched closely.

Another problem can occur when the umbilical cord is connected to the edge rather than the centre of the placenta. This may mean the babies aren't getting enough blood or nutrients. Unfortunately nothing can be done to improve the nutrient and blood supply.

REMEMBER

These complications are not common, and the chance of them happening to you is slim. It is sensible to be aware of the signs so you can seek help if necessary. Don't hesitate to contact your hospital or medical adviser if you have any concerns.

TIPS FOR SURVIVING A TWIN PREGNANCY

- Never hesitate to ring or visit your medical advisers, it is their job (not yours) to decide whether a symptom needs treatment.
- Contact your AMBA or NZMBA group and meet other families with twins.
- Attend playgroups and watch twins in action and chat with their parents.
- Look after yourself – go to bed early and get into comfy bra, clothes and shoes.
- Talk about how you're feeling.
- Do your pelvic floor exercises, perineal massage and take good care of your back.
- Plan to leave work as early as possible.
- Learn as much as you can about breastfeeding during pregnancy – go to a class, see a breastfeeding consultant or watch and talk with other breastfeeding mums of twins.
- Discuss the birth and pain relief with your medical advisers.
- Don't worry about what might go wrong. The odds are on your side that things will all go well.

TIPS FOR PARTNERS

- Tell your partner you love her and that she looks beautiful.
- Spend time talking together about the excitement and about anything that's worrying you.
- Do the housework.
- Organise the children, take them out, give her some time alone.
- Encourage your partner to get as much rest as possible.
- Offer massages or back and foot rubs.
- Do your best to be cheerful and optimistic.
- Know your hospital and arrange transport.
- Listen to her working through her thoughts out loud. Don't feel you need to provide answers.

Safety, cupboards and compost

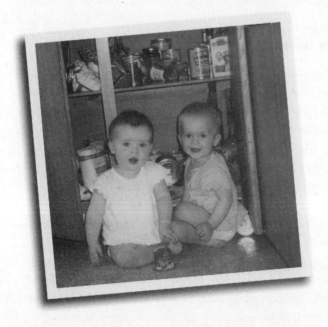

GETTING ORGANISED

GETTING ORGANISED: OUR STORIES

You need rest during a twin pregnancy but you also need to prepare as much as possible for the arrival of your babies. Once they are born you may not have time to do anything other than look after them and twins are more likely to arrive early. This is also the time to take advantage of all offers of help and to plan support for when you're home. Getting organised is also important psychological preparation – it may help you feel more 'ready'.

Katrina: One of the best things I did was sort out all that stuff in the spare room and the junk cupboards – the old letters, the packets of photos waiting for album space, the clothes that are never really worn, my own childhood paraphernalia. Space and structure took on a higher priority.

Louise: I overestimated exactly how much I could organise. A week before my scheduled caesarean at 38 weeks, I had a trailer load of compost delivered on the front driveway. It was still there when the girls celebrated their second birthday (covered in thriving weeds).

Private health cover

Contacting your health insurer now will avoid any misunderstandings later. Let them know you are expecting twins and ask whether two newborns are covered immediately. You may now need family health cover, not singles or couple cover and there may be specific conditions to your contract. Make sure your babies will be covered if one or both are admitted to the special care nursery. Also check what cover you have and ask for a copy of your entitlements in writing.

Check that your private health cover includes ambulance cover – some don't. If not, take out ambulance cover before the birth. It's very expensive to transfer pre-term twins by ambulance.

ANOTHER MUM SAYS 'We had private health cover, which I assumed covered using an ambulance. I later found out it didn't and that only one of my babies was covered for care in the Special Care Nursery.'

ANOTHER MUM SAYS 'I rang my private health company who said we were all covered no matter what. I wrote down the details of the conversation, the time I rang and the person I spoke to. I also asked him to put our conversation in writing, sign it and send it to me. A bill for thousands of dollars arrived for the hospital stay for one of the babies but I had so much evidence of the reassurance I'd been given that I didn't have to pay.'

Your job

If you are working, start thinking about when you'd like to stop or cut down on your hours. If you are planning to return to work within 12 months, you may need to organise childcare while you are pregnant. Demand for childcare centre places is high in some areas and you may need to go on waiting lists. Talk with people about which are the best centres or services then visit them. Your local council will have a complete list of services available.

Preparing older children

ANOTHER MUM SAYS 'My biggest fear was how I would manage twins and my 18-month-old daughter. I was terrified I'd be so busy that she would feel unloved.'

If you have older children, there are many ways to make life easier when your babies arrive.

- Organise others to get to know your older children so they can be given some special time and attention when your babies arrive.
- Arrange where your older children will go when you're in hospital. List contact numbers for: you in hospital, grandparents, friends, school, childcare, doctor, anyone who may need to be contacted.
- Look at the calendar for the few months around your due date and organise any birthday or other presents they may need.
- Organise new routines with older children, showering in the morning or putting their school clothes out at night.
- Buy them a doll or two and play 'babies'.

- Focus on the arrival being their brothers or sisters rather than your new babies.
- Read them stories about a new baby (or two!) arriving in the family.
- Encourage them to talk to the babies in your tummy.
- Encourage special friends to give them special attention.
- Spend time talking with them and reassure them you'll always love them, even if sometimes you will seem busy with the babies.
- Explain that they may need to tell you when they need or want anything.
- Thank them for helping you.
- Accustom them to 'staying' with special family or friends.
- Let them buy a special present for each of the babies.
- Buy a present for the babies to give the older children. It's useful if it's something to keep them amused while visiting you in hospital, like colouring books or a jigsaw.
- When the babies arrive they will receive a lot of attention. To stop your older children feeling left out, always introduce them to admiring strangers.

ANOTHER MUM SAYS   'A girlfriend of mine had identical twin babies as her first 'baby' and she really struggled. When I was expecting my twins I visited her one day and amid the chaos her mother raised her eyebrows at my two-your-old and said to me 'Oh, you poor thing! What a shame you didn't have your twins first up ... you'll have your hands full!' When I eventually had my twins many people commented on how calm and relaxed I seemed even when they were both waiting for my attention. The first few weeks were unbelievably hard and I thought of my friend often. She had never breastfed one, let alone two babies before. She had never experienced sleep deprivation before. She and her husband had never cared for a new baby before. They'd had so much to learn on top of adjusting to their instant family. No wonder she always seemed so stressed and overwhelmed. In retrospect I truly wonder how we would have fared without the confidence and knowledge gained from our first baby. A stressed-out husband and inexperienced mother makes an interesting equation.

Children are a gift but sometimes amid their demands we lose sight of their worth. Often we don't appreciate things until they have gone … like babyhood. My first child revealed to me how quickly babies grow and change. My first baby blossomed into a child in the blink of an eye, so I made a point of slowing down and cherishing my infant twins a little more. This genuinely took effort, as these babies had me running in circles most days. But to stop and cuddle one for no other reason than to just appreciate them was something I had learned from my first child. Equally so, the difficult stages such as the sleepless nights, reflux, teething, etc. were better coped with knowing that this would pass and eventually become a blur in my memory.'

ANOTHER MUM SAYS 'One of the stresses during my twin pregnancy was how my daughter, then two years old, would cope with the massive change in our lives. We'd had such a close and indulgent relationship and I knew her world was about to turn upside down. With an older sibling, there is simply no 'time-out' from being a constant mother. When my husband is not at work he is 'at work' at home. He takes our daughter out on her own to the park and gives me the chance to do the same. I take her to the supermarket on her own as an outing, or I take one of the boys and he takes her and the other boy walking. We're now trying to challenge the dynamic of our little girl and the twins being two separates by giving her time with both boys individually. As the boys get older we're attempting more family outings even though it would be easier for one of us to remain home with the boys. It's important for our daughter to slowly gain an understanding of being patient and tolerant of having two younger brothers and the changes it makes to some experiences. In hindsight, the first few months present few joys for an older sibling. There is constant feeding, irritable and tired parents and little response from the babies other than crying. We probably separated her from this with the help of family and friends. As the babies become responsive to her attempts to make them smile and they laugh and move around she is coming back into the family; sharing special moments rather than us shielding her from the babies. We are learning as we go!'

ANOTHER MUM SAYS   'Make it an absolute family priority to get some free or paid help. If you can afford it, get paid help as it is guilt-free and non-negotiable. Book more help than you think you need, not less. You can use any 'left over' time to do something for yourself. The first year of your babies' lives is not the time to save money. Sell something you don't need, have a pre-baby garage sale or ask your parents for an advance on your inheritance. Even a few hundred dollars worth of help can go a long way to saving your sanity and your marriage.'

Preparing your home for your babies' arrival

- Compile a list of emergency phone numbers and keep them by the phone – doctor, hospital, ambulance, neighbours, Parentline, Australian Breastfeeding Association, La Leche NZ, Lifeline, AMBA, NZMBA, child and family services . . .
- Start buying and borrowing equipment for your babies.
- Scrounge clothes and toys from friends whose babies are older.
- Organise home internet access for emailing friends and shopping online.
- Find out about ringing shopping orders through and having them home delivered.
- Plan your meals ahead of shopping, and make sure you buy all the ingredients so you only shop once.
- When cooking, make double and freeze half so you have ready meals when you arrive home with two babies.
- Ask friends who can cook to drop in some soups and casseroles that you can pop in the freezer. Whip these out when you're starving with no time or energy to cook, either before or after the babies arrive.
- You might decide to unclutter your home. Putting away your knick-knacks temporarily means less time spent dusting. This will also mean less effort 'childproofing' the house when your toddlers are crawling, walking and climbing.
- If you have drawers, cupboards or a spare room containing lots of bits and pieces that need sorting out, you could do it now.
- Start to adjust now to the idea of letting the housework slip. Do things every second day or every second week.

- Consider hiring some help around the house.
- Keep cleaning products in the room where they'll be needed, especially if you have an upstairs bathroom.
- Set up two baby change areas – one at each end of the house.
- Have a mobile change area (a picnic basket with nappies, wipes and creams). Sometimes it's easier to bring the nappy gear to the babies than the babies to the nappy gear.

If you can afford them and don't already have them, consider buying:

Clothes dryer: You will be washing most days, even when the sun doesn't shine, and sometimes it will be difficult to get out to the clothes line. If you only wash when it's sunny, things can quickly get out of hand.

Answering machine or message service: An answering machine means you can still keep in touch with people, even when your hands are full with babies. There will be times when you don't have the desire or energy to talk to people, so it becomes a handy device to 'screen' for important calls.

Portable or 'hands-free' telephone: You will be able to talk more freely on the phone if you can chat with your feet up in front of the TV, in bed or at the clothes line.

Freezer: If you are able to do lots of cooking now, a deep freeze will help you store it.

Microwave: Microwaves are excellent, not just for babies' needs, but for your own instant food requirements. Defrost frozen meals at the last minute.

Dishwasher: If you can stash the dirty dishes away, you feel that things are tidy. And, for some reason men seem to like to pack and unpack dishwashers.

ANOTHER MUM SAYS   'During my pregnancy, I was showered with offers of help for when the twins arrived. Relatives tossed ideas around and grand schemes were formed to assist us when the time came. I was foolishly optimistic that these promises of help would 'fall into place' and that family would stand by their word and 'be there' at a moment's notice. If I were to have my time again, while I was still pregnant I would have organised all offers of help into practical 'concrete' plans by drawing up a four to eight week roster for those wanting to come over and help on a regular basis. This should realistically reflect the time they can actually spare and be available. The roster should target your busiest times, when help is really going to be of assistance. This roster will let family/friends know when they'll be expected and also give you some comeback if they constantly let you down. While this sounds harsh, I found our lack of honest 'demand' caused us to become angry at our families.

Making use of your time

Prepare in advance to spend a couple of weeks with your feet up before the birth. If you find yourself spending time on the couch you could:

- Watch all the movies you taped but never got around to watching.
- Mend the clothes, sew on their missing buttons, patch little tears etc.
- Have a pile of novels handy.
- Address thank you notes in advance.
- Organise friends to pick you up and take you to films or out to lunch during those last couple of weeks.
- Stop and enjoy the feeling of your babies moving inside you.
- Take photos of the pregnant you, including bare-belly shots. People later will want to know 'how big' you got – and you will soon forget!
- Write a 'welcome' letter to your babies or keep a diary of your thoughts to share with your children when they're older.
- List all the possible names for your babies.
- Have some special time with your partner. Do something out of the ordinary whether it's going to the theatre or having a picnic by the beach.

Pack your hospital bag

If you pack your hospital bag sooner rather than later, it'll be ready to go when you are. You may want to pack:

- nighties and pyjamas that allow easy access for breastfeeding two at a time
- slippers and dressing gown
- maternity bras
- breast pads (to absorb the leaks)
- knickers – disposable as well as normal
- maternity pads – at least three packs
- comfortable (loose!) clothes for lounging around hospital
- a good barrier cream for your hands. You'll be washing them constantly once the babies arrive.
- CDs – music to scream by . . .
- list of who to phone and their number – in order of priority
- your 'no visitors' signs
- this book and maybe others
- a blank paged book and a pen if you want to start a diary or keep notes
- champagne and plastic cups to celebrate!
- clothes and nappies to bring your babies home in. Check with your hospital whether it provides clothes for baby during hospital stay.

Other things to grab on your way out the door are:

- toiletries, make-up and hair dryer
- some cash
- camera – including batteries and film. Borrow a Polaroid if you can for some instant shots.
- Medicare card, healthcare card

Most hospitals have a shop that stocks the essentials if you forget or run out.

Equipment

In addition to plenty of love, all your newborn babies are really going to need is something to eat, somewhere to sleep, and clothes to wear.

This is a simple reminder that you don't need to spend a fortune. Baby shops stock all sorts of gorgeous things that, although tempting, are often unnecessary and sometimes expensive or impractical. You don't need two of everything either; you might start with one of some things and adopt a wait and see approach.

What will they eat? Be prepared. Where and when will they sleep? Be prepared.

Cots

Only buy cots that conform to the Australian and New Zealand Standards for household use (AS/NZS 2172). These standards do not permit gaps where a child's head or body could become trapped or bits that stick out that could snag a child's clothing and cause strangulation.

Make sure the cots you buy have:
- vertical bars no further apart than eight centimetres so baby can't wedge his or her head in between
- a firm and fitting mattress, with no more than a two centimetre gap between the mattress and the side of the cot
- no more than two legs with castors or castors which have brakes on them
- at least half a metre between the top of the cot and the top of the mattress (on the lowest possible base)
- surfaces which are free of any footholds or toeholds, such as heart-shaped cut-outs, or 'wood-turned' features
- drop-down sides or a height-adjustable mattress

Most cot injuries occur when children fall while trying to climb out of cots. Once they start climbing out, they have outgrown their cot and it's time to move them to a bed.

Never use an old portable cot without the loud, clicking mechanism on its sides. Several babies have died over the last five years in Australia when their older model portable cot collapsed at the sides and caught their necks and suffocated them. If in doubt about the age and design of the portable cot, don't use it.

A booklet called 'Keeping Baby Safe – A Guide to Nursery Furniture' is available from Consumer Affairs, Department of Fair Trading.

Katrina: We put the girls in one cot near the window so that they could admire the view but we made sure curtain cords were out of their reach. One of the girls was more alert so we faced her away from the door. Once they were in separate cots we positioned them parallel about a metre apart so that they could see, but not touch, each other. It seemed important to them to know that they were both going to bed, not just one.

Louise: Our cots had solid ends and were placed end to end, largely because of the design restrictions of the room. They would throw toys over to each other and stand up to see and talk to each other.

Bedding

You will need:

- Mattress protectors.
- Three sheets per cot is a good start, you don't have to use top sheets. If you have 'chucky' babies, you can put a cloth nappy down, but there still may be days where you change the linen more than once. Choose sheets that fit as cot sizes vary.
- Two blankets per baby during the colder months.
- If it's summer and you don't have flyscreens on the windows, or if you live in a tropical or insect-prone area, mosquito nets can be useful.

TIPS ABOUT BEDDING

- Cot bumpers and pillows are unsafe for children under two years of age.
- Cot mattress sizes vary. Make sure the mattress fits the cot snugly so that heads can't be caught between the cot and mattress and cause suffocation.
- It is often cheaper to purchase single bed sized sheets and blankets and either creatively fold them under the mattress or cut and sew them to fit two cots.

Bath

A baby bath isn't essential. Setting up a bathing area on your kitchen table or bench can be time and energy consuming. You may find the laundry tub or the big bath more convenient, but remember that it's best for your well-being to bathe your babies at a height that is kind to your back. Don't lift a baby bath full of water by yourself – get help to tip it out. The various inserts that offer baby support in the baby bath aren't necessary, they grow out of them quickly and you may find they get in your way. You needn't bathe your babies every day, just a daily wipe down and a bath every second or third day is fine.

Once your babies are sitting up, at least one bath ring seat is useful so that when both babies are in the bath, one is secure in the seat while you're washing the other. Of course, even in a bath ring, babies still must be supervised, but it means you don't have to 'hold-down' two babies at once! Once they're standing up, they like to practise while in the bath. Make sure you have a rubber mat to provide some grip at the base of the bath, but discourage them from standing. It's a bit hazardous.

You will need four bath towels, multiple flannels and a suitable soap-free bath product.

> **MAKE THIS A HABIT**
> Always empty the bath before you leave the bathroom.
> Make it a habit before your toddler leans over and falls in.

Change table

Some parents never use a change table, others use one, while some parents of twins have two. As with everything else it's a personal choice. A portable change table is handy if you're setting up a 'baby bathing station' in the kitchen, laundry or bathroom. A shelf nearby is handy for nappies, wipes, clothes and cream. A moveable trolley on wheels is ideal to hold nappies, wipes, cream etc. and can be wheeled around to change babies in their bassinette, cot or wherever. Have a bin nearby and some dustbin bags handy too.

Other parents of twins recommend a large solid table in the nursery. It can be used for changing, bathing and storage of some clothes and linen so they're handy when needed.

Alternatively, you can buy a thick changing pad with raised sides, which is used on a bed or chest of drawers.

Never leave a child alone on a change table because they can fall off.

ANOTHER MUM SAYS 'I'm sure the change table helped save my back. If I'd been on the floor all the time, I'd have been bending more. The change table enabled everything to be placed within my comfortable reach.'

ANOTHER MUM SAYS 'We used a wobbly change table for 18 months, then in order to get some space back we got rid of it and started to change them on the spare bed or on the floor. This was just fine once they were bigger, also because they often insisted on being changed whilst standing up.'

Baby monitors

Whether you need a baby monitor often depends on the design of your house, or the noise levels in your home. For some parents it gives a feeling of reassurance. If you spend a lot of time hanging washing on the line, or gardening, then you may find a baby monitor useful.

Rockers and bouncinettes

Think about these things:

- One for each baby is handy.
- It is somewhere to pop your babies when they're awake but aren't being cuddled or spending time on the floor.
- Some babies will nap in their rockers.
- You can move babies around the house/yard to be near you.
- You can prop a baby in a rocker to bottle-feed.
- When breastfeeding you can place your babies on rockers while you seat yourself and get comfortable, then lift them from their rocker up to you.
- They are great to take out when visiting.
- Some portable car capsules double as a baby rocker. These are not to lift your baby out of with one hand. An open bouncinette or rocker is better when you're single-handed.
- Never place your rockers on a table, always on the floor. If there are toddlers or animals around, keep a close eye to make sure your babies are safe.
- Strap babies in. Wherever there are straps, use them.

Furniture in your babies' bedroom

A large set of drawers and a wardrobe can be very useful. Once mobile, your babies will probably be into small sets of drawers and pulling everything off bookshelves. This is useful if you want them to be able to get at their toys but it's easier to keep things a bit tidy if you have wardrobe doors and drawers a toddler can't open.

If you have room, a spare bed in the babies' room is invaluable as a place to read stories to them, give them a morning feed or sleep near them without disturbing your partner. A rocking chair or armchair to sit and feed or cuddle your babies in their bedroom can also be useful.

What will they wear?

If you have older children your babies might wear clothes you already have. Friends and family are often generous when twins are born. You may be given both new and used clothes and equipment. If you start with the basics, you can add later at sale time. The following list should be enough for your babies, depending on the season:

- 8 singlets
- 12 nighties (excellent for easy bottom access) or 12 jumpsuits (zips are a great time-saver, press studs are more time consuming) or 12 separate tops and bottoms
- 6 cardigans/jackets/fleecy tops
- 4 brushed cotton wraps for winter babies or 4 cotton or gauze wraps for summer
- 4 hats
- 8 pairs of socks
- plenty of bibs

All-in-one outfits make baby handling easy for parents juggling two wrigglers, however separates are also useful as you only need to change one half of the baby if they are sick on their top or soil their bottoms. Pants with foot enclosures attached are great. Socks and booties are kicked off and lost all the time, all-in-ones keep those toes warm. Little crib shoes help keep the socks on but can be time-consuming to get on and off four feet!

Sizes of clothes vary greatly and like adult clothes, vary between brands. Most full term babies are 00. Twins tend to be 38 weeks or earlier and are usually a bit smaller, so 000 is often the best fit. They do tend to grow out of 000 quickly and you get more use from 00. You can always send someone out to buy smaller or larger gear if needed.

> **A GENERAL GUIDE TO SIZING**
> 000 – birth to 3 months
> 00 – 3 to 6 months
> 0 – 6 to12 months

In the past, pre-term babies would often be dressed in dolls clothes but a good range of 0000 and 00000 clothes is now available if you find you need them. Your local AMBA or NZMBA club may also have some pre-term clothes you can buy or borrow.

Dressing your babies the same

Little babies neither know nor care whether they're dressed differently or the same, but it can influence the way others see them. It helps others to tell them apart if they are dressed differently – even if they're not identical. If they are dressed the same, it encourages people to treat them as one entity. Many parents of twins dress their babies in variations on a theme. For example, the same outfit in different colours or both in different types of overalls. Once twins are older they may insist on being dressed the same or differently. Once they can choose, it's fine to let them.

ANOTHER MUM SAYS   'I swore I would not dress my twins the same. I felt that as identical twins they would have enough of an identity crisis, and I didn't want to add to the fact. When they were born we were given so many gorgeous matching outfits, occasionally I couldn't resist having a matching pair. We did our best to stick to a rule, one in the pink and one in yellow. This helped everyone else know who was who, without having to think too hard about it.'

Nappies

Cloth or disposable? This is the question most prospective parents ask. Whichever you use, there will be an awful lot of them and your babies will be in them for about three years. With twins, you will probably use more than 14 000 nappies.

The Australian Consumer Association's *Choice* magazine published a study in August 1999 comparing cost, and concluded that cloth nappies are much cheaper than disposables. The study quoted the NSW Environment Protection Authority saying that taking into account the water, bleach and energy used to launder cloth nappies, there is no clear environmental advantage between the two. *Choice* goes on to say that disposable nappies make up about one per cent of landfill.

Some parents use cloth nappies all the time, either through a nappy wash service or washing and drying them themselves. Some parents always use disposable nappies. Others use cloth during the day, and disposables at night or when travelling. Childcare centres often want children to arrive and go home wearing disposables but will put them in cloth nappies in between.

> (ANOTHER MUM SAYS) 'I had a lot of well-meaning advice from mothers who hadn't had twins, about how cloth nappies really aren't that much bother and how they can soak overnight, you just need to rinse them and hang them out. I told them that I'd be quite happy to use cloth nappies if they would pick the dirty ones up and drop clean ones off twice a week.'

Cloth nappies

You will need around 60 cloth nappies: 20 per day, 20 in the wash and 20 in the cupboard. You'll need pins, fasteners, liners, waterproof pants, two nappy buckets and sanitising nappy-soak powder. Remember to keep the lids of nappy buckets firmly in place, and out of reach, so that once babies are on the move, there's no risk of drowning.

ADVANTAGES OF CLOTH NAPPIES
- They are possibly better for the environment.
- They are cheaper than disposables.

DISADVANTAGES OF CLOTH NAPPIES
- They need to be changed more often as they're not as absorbent. More moisture against the skin means more nappy rash.
- Changing the nappy and the waterproof pants, and perhaps clothes, more often increases your workload.
- Fussing with pins and fasteners can become difficult with squirmy toddlers.
- Washing cloth nappies is time consuming. They need to be soaked then washed or rinsed, then hung on the line or put in the drier.

Disposable nappies

Your newborns will each use about eight nappies a day. As they get older this number will drop. You'll probably try a few different brands to find the best value for money for your babies – some babies get a lot wetter than others, some have more squirty poo than others. If you plan to use disposable nappies, it is still worth having a dozen or so cloth nappies in the house. They come in very handy as 'spew rags', laying down under baby and dribble protectors for your clothes. You need to dispose of your dirty nappies responsibly: tie them in old plastic shopping bags or you can buy little perfumed bags to pop them in. You can also use a lined rubbish bin with a tight fitting lid. You can even buy nappy disposal equipment that works like a sausage machine individually wrapping each soiled nappy!

ADVANTAGES OF DISPOSABLE NAPPIES
- Twin mums have less spare time and energy so can find disposables much easier to use.
- They're more absorbent so don't need to be changed as often
- Less leakage onto clothes.
- Paper-lined disposable nappies breathe, decreasing the chance of nappy rash.
- Normal and seconds can be purchased and delivered direct from the factory to your door. These are all the popular brands and at much cheaper prices than supermarkets. Metropolitan and some regional areas offer this service. Often you can place these orders online.

DISADVANTAGES OF DISPOSABLE NAPPIES

- Toilet training happens later, as disposables are more comfortable and children have less incentive to get out of them.
- Some disposables increase nappy rash on sensitive skin.
- Some parents believe the chemicals in disposables aren't good for young babies.
- They're more expensive than cloth but cost about the same as a nappy wash service.
- When disposing of them, remember that poos are supposed to be flushed down the toilet, but this is tricky initially when it's all so runny.
- Landfill.
- The trees, the trees ...

Nappy wash service

The disadvantages are the same as those above for cloth nappies except a service will save you the time and bother of soaking and washing nappies. You can often choose between folded nappies or fold your own. If the service is available in your area, the cost of cloth nappy wash services is comparable to purchasing disposables. A nappy wash pick-up and delivery service is sometimes given as a gift. Some parents of twins love it others prefer disposables because of the need to change cloths and clothes more frequently.

> (ANOTHER MUM SAYS) 'I tried to use a nappy wash service, but it didn't suit me. Even with someone picking up and dropping them off I still had to remember to put them out the night before pick-up, fold them when they arrived and I seemed to do nothing but change nappies as they got wet so quickly. I also hated having stinky, dirty nappies hanging around the house.'

Wipes

There is also the cloth versus disposable argument when it comes to wiping your babies' bums. You're the best person to decide what suits you and your family, as each option has its pros and cons.

Cloth (flannel)

Flannels are cheaper, and the fabric is better for babies' bottoms than paper products. They do need soaking and washing. The cloths need to be rinsed in warm water before you change the baby's nappy, and by the time you're ready to change the second baby, warm cloths have turned cold.

Disposable wipes

They are instantly on hand and ready to use at all times, and don't need washing – just throwing out. Although they are more expensive than the cloth option, they come in handy for wiping faces and hands when you're not at home. Remember though that paper products can be rougher on babies bottoms and cause chafing on some babies.

Cotton wool or tissues with baby cream/lotion

Both are gentle on the skin, and clean thoroughly in all the creases. You can flush tissues easily down the loo. Nappy lotions double as protective creams. It is, however, likely to be messy, and might be difficult to manage with two wriggling bubs. It's also a potentially costly option.

Car

If you don't have a car or a licence, then this may be the right time to get them. It's difficult to manage on public transport with a twin pram. Buses and trams are impossible, but many metropolitan trains cater for disabled passengers, and can accommodate parents with twin prams. Most taxi services offer front facing baby seats (not capsules), and you can book cabs with two seats if you book in advance. Walking your babies is great, but doing this all the time depends on the weather and living near all the services you will need.

Once babies are around four months old, toys are useful in the car, along with 'linking-rings' from which to suspend toys so they remain an entertaining fixture.

Car capsules/seats

Keep your children safe when you travel by car by always using approved child restraints which meet the Australian and New Zealand standards (AS/NZS 1754). The law holds the driver responsible for appropriately restraining children under 16 years of age.

The dual capsule/car seat systems are very useful but only if you have a big car like a Ford Falcon, Holden Commodore or Mitsubishi Magna. Most other cars do not have enough room for them. Make sure you consult with staff at the 'expert fitting station' before purchasing seats to make sure they will fit in your car. While the label might claim that the capsule will fit into all models of cars, this is often only true if it's placed in the middle of the rear seat. This is fine if you only need one capsule. With two capsules, you'll be putting at least one behind a front seat, and many seemingly large cars don't have the room for this.

Capsules that can be easily removed from the car and have a carry-handle can be useful because you can remove sleeping babies into or out of the car without waking them. Remember that they are meant for use in the car – they are quite heavy and carrying them is not good for your back. Don't leave a baby in a capsule on the driveway or between parked cars – they have been known to get run over.

If buying a restraint or child seat second-hand, make sure the seat has not been in an accident and that there are no structural cracks or deficiencies and that it still has the right straps and anchor bolts.

Instead of buying, you can often hire child seats through your local council, maternal and child health centre, some hospitals and private hire companies. Organise this during your pregnancy to make sure two are available at the same time.

Make sure you have the seats installed correctly. You may need additional straps and anchor bolts. If you can, take advantage of the qualified restraint fitting stations. Correct installation and use includes:

- The baby restraints should be anchored firmly to the car using the top tether strap.
- The seat belt should be attached exactly as shown in the instructions.
- The securing straps should not be slack. Check every time you use them.
- The shoulder straps should be just above your babies' shoulders or at shoulder height.
- The harness must be buckled firmly around the babies, you should just be able to squeeze a finger in between baby and belt.

Baby size	Car seat type
Up to 9 kg–12 kg* and 700 mm–850 mm long (up to around six months)	Rear-facing infant restraint/ capsule
8–19 kg (approx. six months to four years)	Front-facing child seat
14–32 kg (four years to eight years)	Child harness with lap/sash or lap-only belt (used with booster seat between 14–26 kg)

* Limits vary so check the weight marked on the restraint

Pram/stroller

Many AMBA and NZMBA clubs provide a pram-hire service for a nominal fee. This enables you to try before you buy. A popular option is to hire the baby-friendly pram which is only used for the first few months before you buy a parent-friendly car-boot-fitting stroller.

FEATURES TO LOOK FOR IN YOUR TWIN PRAM/STROLLER

- It complies with the Australian Standard (AS/NZS 2088).
- It's not too heavy to lug into the boot and out and in and out ...
- Bigger wheels are best – they give you more momentum, so you use less force.
- Bigger shopping trays are best – you will be carrying a lot of baby gear when you go out, or you can use the pram tray to carry groceries home.
- It's weather proof, with rain, wind and sun covers (universal covers are available separately if not sold with the pram).
- It's easy to assemble with the flick of a wrist.
- It fits in your car boot easily.
- The handle is the right height for you so you're not stooping as you push.
- Full handles, rather than 'umbrella' handles, can help when lifting the pram up curbs and steps.
- It has proper five point baby restraints, including crotch strap and straps that go over both shoulders and around the waist.

Most new side-by-side models are a slimmer design and fit through most doors. The tandem models with seats in front of each other can be difficult to turn when full and a potential traffic hazard when the front baby can see the car coming before you can! Most tandem prams are designed for an older toddler and a new baby, rather than twins. The front seat often doesn't recline completely without squashing the leg room of the back passenger.

If you have older children who still require a pram or stroller seat, you may be able to hire what you need through your AMBA or NZMBA branch. Booster seats are available on some double prams like the Emmaljunga Double Grizzly that can hold up to four children. The Triton Trekker has an attachable toddler seat which goes low on the front of the buggy so babies in the rear can still see. 'Mountain Buggy' makes a triple jogger-type pram. There may be others that you can investigate further at the pram shop. Boogie board attachments are another option for your toddler to hitch a ride.

> **TIPS FOR PUSHING A DOUBLE PRAM**
> Keep your elbows bent – it's easier.

Hammocks/swings

For your babies, being rock, rock, rocked is often a soothing alternative to being in your arms. Hammocks and swings come in windup or electric designs or just old-fashioned manual where you give them the odd push to keep them swinging. Many parents of unsettled babies insist swings are life-savers. One may be enough. They can be bought or hired from your AMBA or NZMBA branch.

ANOTHER MUM SAYS 'One of our girls spent between 5 and 9 p.m. in the swing every night for the first six months of her life. She was so unsettled at that time of day and it was the only thing that calmed her. We wound up the swing, it rocked for 45 minutes then stopped, she'd start screaming and we'd wind it up again. Silence.'

Playpens

Some parents find playpens a useful and safe place to put the babies while they dash to the loo or to answer the front door. A playpen can also provide a safe haven from a jealous older sibling, or give parents a place to sit in while doing baby unfriendly activities (sewing!). Once mobile, babies may protest at their imprisonment in a playpen. Twins also work in cahoots to escape, with one lifting the playpen while the other crawls out. Port-a-cots have 'floors' and can make suitable playpens.

> ANOTHER MUM SAYS   'I kept the ironing board set up in the playpen for 18 months (until they could push the playpen around the room). I thought it would save setting the ironing board up all the time, but I only used the iron twice!'

Highchairs

You don't need highchairs until around six months, when babies are sitting up. The two main features to look for in a highchair are that it is easy to clean and has a safety harness which includes a crotch strap.

An alternative to highchairs are chairs that clamp onto the dining table. They save space and are more portable. Check first that they will fit your table and that your table is sufficiently sturdy. It is often difficult to find two highchairs when eating out. However, when out, you can usually feed solids to your babies while they're sitting in their stroller. Before long, they'll want to sit on the 'big chairs' like you.

Baby bouncers/Jolly Jumpers

Babies delight in bouncing up and down in these seats that hang from a doorframe. Your twins will love a bouncer each in their own doorway so they can see each other. These are only useful from about six months when babies can hold their heads up firmly. Bouncers are not recommended for prolonged use but used wisely they are fine as long as they are put up safely. It is a lot of effort to hook them up and strap them in for such a short time. Depending on the style and the door, some have to be attached to a hook which is permanently screwed to the doorframe. If in doubt, get professional advice from a physio or from your maternal child health centre.

(ANOTHER MUM SAYS) 'We hardly used it because it was so much effort. We had one and had to adjust it for each baby because they were two different sizes. By the time they'd both had a turn I was exhausted. Even if we'd had two Jolly Jumpers I would still have found it too much trouble.'

Baby walkers

The latest research on baby walkers indicates they provide no benefit, can hinder walking development and that they are an unacceptable risk. The Child Safety Report by Mater Hospital's Injury Surveillance Unit in Brisbane says they should not be used under any circumstances. However, if you do decide to use them, make sure any stairs or uneven floor levels are barricaded off with a childproof gate or similar.

Toys

You'll need a few soft toys, rattles, mobiles, blocks with bells in them etc. while your babies are very little. At about three to four months you will all enjoy an activity gym which the babies lie under. Two babies will fit under most styles. Toys playing simple musical tunes (musical mobiles, music boxes etc.) can provide distracting entertainment for young babies.

Moving your babies around the house to see a different view of the world or to watch you doing a range of activities or just watching each other will provide them with plenty of stimulation for their first months of life.

Swap toys with friends and relatives or join a local toy library. Kitchen utensils can make great toys, too.

Toy boxes

Avoid toy boxes with heavy hinged lids. Babies can crawl inside and get stuck or suffocate. If you do have one of these, then drill air holes in the top and at the back and fit rubber or stoppers that allow a gap when the lid is closed.

Other items you may find useful

- Dummies.
- Night-light – you don't want to turn on the bright nursery light when checking babies in the night. Replacing a clear globe with a blue or green 'party' globe is an effective night-light. Or you could install a dimmer, use the hall light or a small night-light.
- Nappy bag – either a specially designed change bag or just include a change mat in your everyday backpack.
- Puddle feeders – wrap-around 'smock style' long sleeved plastic bibs – great when you're introducing solids and wanting to protect clothes. You just wipe or rinse all the gunk off then leave the smock to dry before the next meal. These are available from the Australian Breastfeeding Association.
- Dribble bibs – small plastic-backed collar bibs designed to protect babies' clothes and skin from dribble while not disguising that gorgeous outfit.
- Dribble-proof singlets and spencers, that keep moisture away from your babies' skin.
- Sleeping bags – a fleecy-lined bag with sleeves. Keep your babies warm in winter when they start kicking off their blankets. Useful from about six months to when they're standing (around 12 months)
- Pram sack – a hooded bag for winter babies in their pram. It will keep a baby warm without the effort of mittens, hats, rugs etc. Very cosy but not safe for bed. An 'indulgent' purchase useful for up to four months.
- Slings/pouches – useful to carry an unsettled baby around the house with you while you do some jobs. Get two if there is an adult per baby, but don't try and wear two slings at a time. Look after your back because you will need it later.
- Baby backpack – sophisticated light metal ones carry a baby that is old enough to hold its head up. Men seem to love them. Some of them convert into a stand-alone seat so you can seat your baby next to you while you sit and have a coffee. You'll need somewhere for the other baby too, so use when you have one in a single pusher or someone else to carry them.

- Port-a-cot/s – good for travelling, staying overnight, or even to take to a friend's for dinner so the babies can still sleep comfortably while you socialise. You can buy a large port-a-cot to accommodate two young babies, but as they get older you would need two. Check that the large one or two smaller ones will still fit in your car, along with the pram and everything else. Also check that port-a-cots conform to Australian standards and check their weight limits.

Money-saving tips

The expense of twins can be greater than one baby largely because you don't necessarily hand things down from one baby to the next. There can be a lot of pressure to spend big on your babies.

You will probably be given presents following their birth. People are generous when it comes to twins. Don't rush out and buy lots of things – just get the basics. You don't need anything new for your babies. Borrow items that are used for a short time, like baby baths, rockers etc. from friends or family who have had babies. Buy second-hand, always checking goods meet Australian and New Zealand Safety Standards. Good sources of second-hand equipment are:

- the trading magazines or newspaper classifieds
- other AMBA and NZMBA members who advertise in your branch newsletter
- school fetes, markets, op shops and charity stores
- garage sales
- second-hand baby equipment shops where parents sell baby gear on consignment. They're a great source for toys, books and videos.

To start with, just purchase a nappy rash ointment (zinc and castor oil cream is very effective) and some soap-free cleanser for the baby bath. You will get sample packs of various things in hospital. You will soon work out what you do really need. Buy nappies and wipes in bulk from a factory outlet.

You don't need a lot of toys until at least after four months. Most sub-urbs have toy libraries with only a token joining fee and one hour 'duty' a school term. Beware of toys with lots of detachable little bits and pieces that keep you searching for days, so you don't have to pay a fine. Lots of books suitable for babies, toddlers and parents can be borrowed from your local library.

Have a garage sale to raise money. You will be amazed by what sells – magazines, books, fabric remnants, clothes, cassette tapes. It's a good chance to make a bit of cash for things you may have otherwise thrown out, given away or stored unnecessarily.

Encourage family, friends and colleagues to chip in for baby store vouchers so you can buy necessities rather than receive luxuries. Start sewing and knitting (not booties) – with all your spare time!

Assess your family budget. Do you need to refinance your mortgage? What costs can you reduce? How can you generate additional income? If one parent is staying at home for a while, you'll probably receive Family Payments from the Family Assistance Office. Australian and New Zealand governments also offer a childcare rebate which makes childcare a more affordable option.

Safety issues

Safety awareness is even more important when you have twins. This is mainly because it is more difficult to watch two or more active crawlers who have no sense of fear or danger. Twins tend to copy each other and encourage each other to be more daring. The greater strength of two, their sense of co-operation and their eagerness to explore the world makes constant supervision necessary but impossible.

Private homes are the most likely place children will be injured. The main dangers are drowning, suffocation, burns, falls and poisoning. Most injuries can be prevented by simple means, so save yourself a lot of worry by removing any hazards.

If you have older children, you will probably have already done a lot of childproofing. However once you're busy with twins, you will not always be able to keep your eye on older children so you need to ensure everything is childproofed. Explore your house now for potential structural changes that should be done in advance and take the following safety precautions now rather than later.

Inside

- Keep a list of emergency numbers near your phone and know the location of your nearest hospital emergency section.
- Install fire alarms and check they are working.
- Make sure any nursery items you purchase meet the Australian and New Zealand Safety Standards.
- Arrange for an electrician to install a circuit breaker in your fuse box to prevent electrocution. Buy safety plugs for power points.
- Have a fire extinguisher and fire blanket handy.
- Get a sturdy safety screen around fireplaces or 'stove' heaters. Get rid of radiators or put sturdy guards around them.
- Put valuable items away or up and out of reach, including TV/video, stereo and precious breakables.
- Rearrange cupboards and drawers throughout the house. Knives, plastic bags, medicines, cleaning products and toiletries should be either locked away or completely inaccessible. Remember that your babies will grow to learn how to open doors, scale shelves and climb kitchen benches.
- Get placemats and store your tablecloths with the mothballs. Babies like to pull down on them and everything else.
- From an early age your babies will put anything small in their mouth so make sure buttons, pins, batteries and small toys belonging to an older child are well out of reach.
- Keep electrical appliances and their cords well away from bench edges.
- Tie up cords to curtains and blinds so babies can't access them and strangle themselves.
- Always stand saucepans on the stove so that handles point to the centre or back.
- Bookshelves and items with height need to be solid so that children can't pull them down on themselves. You may choose to bracket them against the wall. If you love your books put them out of reach for now. Your children might enjoy ripping them to shreds.
- Windows and doors should be secured to prevent children from opening them and climbing out – this is especially important if you have rooms upstairs.
- Glass doors are a hazard. If they're not made of safety glass, a safety film is available.

Outside

- If you have pets that are used to being around the house, think about re-training them to live outside or elsewhere! Animals can be a risk to babies and small children and their water bowls are a potential drowning hazard.
- Remove poisonous plants from parts of the garden your children will access. These include azaleas, daffodils, wisteria, oleander, ferns, poinsettia, daphne, arum and calla lilies, lantana, potato vine, foxglove, golden dewdrop, cape lilac, angel's trumpet, castor oil plant, cestrum, cotoneaster, cycad.
- Fix fences or railings that have vertical railings more than 8 cm apart. Are the fences climbable? If so, how can you change that?
- Your swimming pool should be fenced. Securely cover any ponds, birdbaths, fishbowls, drains or other 'pools' of water. Garden furniture needs to be super heavy, out of reach or bolted down so it can't be used to climb pool fences.
- Enclose or secure access to upper storey decks and verandahs.

Increasing your own safety

Now is not the time for either parent to try abseiling, skiing or skydiving. Look after yourselves because you need to be fit and available for the task ahead. It's just as important to think about your own safety. What do you want or need to feel safe? For example:

- Install security screen doors and/or windows so that you can have airflow while still feeling safe at home.
- Put a rubber mat in your shower or bath.
- Place rubber backing under mats on floorboards or tiles.
- Do your stairs need a railing for additional support?

TIPS FOR GETTING ORGANISED

- Find out about getting things home-delivered.
- De-clutter your home.
- Scrounge, borrow or buy second-hand.
- Cook and freeze nutritious meals.
- Go to antenatal classes.
- Get your finances organised.

TIPS FOR PARTNERS

- Do as much as possible around the house.
- If you don't already know how, learn to cook.
- Arrange some special time together.
- Arrange and install the baby restraints in the car.
- Give some special time to your older children.
- Go to antenatal classes.
- Childproof your yard and home.

How will they get out?

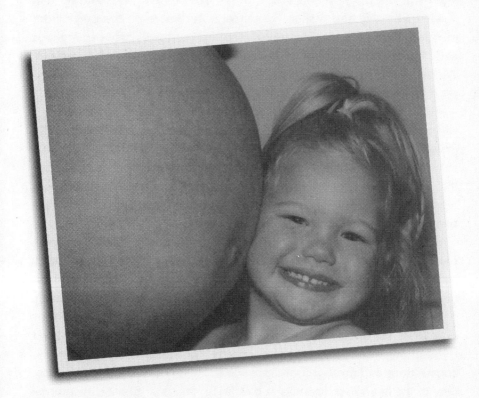

BIRTH

BIRTH: OUR STORIES

It's common for parents, particularly first time parents, to focus on the birth itself. We look forward to meeting our babies, but with some trepidation as to the circumstances. Falling in love with two babies at once may be different to how you imagined. Being prepared, and talking and thinking about what might happen, can ease some of your fear and strengthen your anticipation.

Katrina: At my 36 week obstetrician appointment everything looked good. The babies were head down, but I had no sign that birth was imminent. The next day I felt as ready as I'd ever be. I was feeling some pressure and a tightening that made me think it would happen sooner rather than later, then that night in bed it started. Water trickled from my vagina and I was hopping up and down to the loo, I thought my bladder had finally given way and wished I'd concentrated more on the pelvic floor muscles. When the trickling didn't stop, I put a towel between my legs and rang the hospital. They suggested we come in and get checked out. We packed a bag half-heartedly, thinking it was a false alarm for sure and we'd be back home in an hour. We had no idea.

At 2.30 a.m. we were told we would have these babies by lunchtime, I was already three centimetres dilated. We were excited and I wished I'd packed the CDs after all. Then the water started to gush and the contractions began. I was able to push my feet onto the bed end and 'breathe' through the pain. I was on the bed all this time. I was so big that walking was a problem. Some machines were wheeled in to monitor the babies' heartbeats through belts wrapped around my belly.

By 7a.m. I was 10 cm dilated and although the contractions were more painful, they were still manageable. My sister arrived. A theatre nurse by profession, she was a great help through the birth. Her expertise and sisterly support made for the right combination for my second birth partner.

The anaesthetist was called in and gave me the epidural. I lay on my side while he put a needle into my back. Thoughts of paralysis went through my mind. Then everything pretty well stopped. I could feel the contractions and my legs, but there was never any sense or urge to push. One of the heart monitors wasn't picking up one heartbeat so an internal monitor was positioned. I didn't feel it being put through my vagina. I went to the loo but needed assistance to get there because my legs were like jelly. I wasn't managing to pee so it was decided I should have a catheter. It was inserted quickly and drained away bucket loads helping me feel more comfortable.

The contractions continued but nothing else was happening. Lunchtime arrived and I didn't have my babies. The obstetrician suggested a caesarean. From what I'd read and heard, I thought a caesarean meant a much more difficult recovery and I didn't want one unless absolutely necessary. I asked for some time and said I'd walk around so gravity could do its job. The epidural and various monitors and epidural drips made it tricky to stand up so I didn't venture further than next to the bed. Cold washers on my forehead and hot packs against my back were a big help.

I was glad I had two support people. It meant one could go to the loo or grab coffee or food while the other held my hand. It also lightened the mood. My sister's nursing training meant she was able to explain a lot of the medical aspects to me. She was reassuring and stopped Brad and me from worrying about what was happening.

I still had no pushing urge or sensation. Twin two's heartbeat was showing signs of distress. My obstetrician checked me internally and said he could feel the head but also what he thought was a hand. He thought that a head and arm were trying to come out together and it was unlikely this would happen. With signs of distress he thought it best to proceed with the caesar. I agreed, as it meant my babies would be OK. I was wheeled to surgery straightaway. We were told one guest only so I had to say goodbye to my sister. Brad was lead away to don the theatre robes and mask. I remember questions from hospital staff – any allergies all that sort of stuff. The nurse assisting me was a mother of twins. She told me how gorgeous her girls were. I complimented the anaesthetist on his beautiful, bright blue eyes. I felt at peace and deliriously happy.

It took a big effort to lift me from the bed onto the theatre table. I was shaking with cold and my teeth were chattering. The obstetrician was shaving the top of my pubic hair with an electric razor. My sister was there after all … they let her in, yippee! There were about six staff in the room and a tall screen in front of me so I couldn't see the work on my belly. My husband and sister were each holding a hand and reassuring me that everything was OK. I could feel the incision – not any pain, just the sensation. I could also feel the obstetrician pulling and tugging – very weird. At 3.59 p.m. my first baby girl was born. I burst into tears. Ella Hart was quickly whipped up by staff and taken over to the crib. My first glimpse of her was with staff attending her while she was crying in the crib. We could see her right leg up over her head and thought she was so clever – our little ballerina. Then it became clear that this wasn't quite right. The pediatrician was checking her out and put the leg back into position and corrected her knee. At 4.02 p.m. Charlotte Rose was born. Brad accepted the invitation to cut the cord. Charlotte needed oxygen and extra attention. There was some level of concern on the faces of the staff. I kept asking, 'Is my baby all right, is she all right?' It was very quiet. No one was answering. Brad said reassuring things like 'She'll be OK, darling, the best people are looking after her.' Ella Hart was rugged up and placed in my arms for a quick cuddle. She was beautiful and perfect. It was an overwhelmingly magical moment.

We were worried about Charlotte. I couldn't see her. They said she was getting some oxygen. I was asking for my baby. After a long five minutes she was in my arms. Already asleep and so adorable – just like her sister, and both just like their dad.

We had to hand the babies back and I was wheeled away to recovery alone. There a male nurse looked after me. I was thirsty and he brought me the dozen or so glasses of water I requested. I was there for an hour while he monitored my blood pressure and bleeding, and changed my pads. I was still freezing, apparently a side-effect of the anaesthesia. He gave me snugly warm blankets from the oven. I couldn't stop talking to the nurse … I wanted to know everything about him. Suddenly he was somebody's baby and I loved him.

I was wheeled out again, backwards down the corridors and ended up throwing up all the water I just drank. I was taken to Brad and my sister who had been in the hospital café madly ringing people with the news. I was wheeled into the Special Care Nursery where we joined our babies. All I wanted was sleep but two nurses were holding the babies to my breasts and cameras were snapping away. This really shocked me, I could barely keep my eyes open … I hadn't slept for 32 hours.

For about one minute I was disappointed that I hadn't had a 'natural' birth. I knew it was unlikely I'd have any more children, so I was never going to experience a vaginal birth. I knew the most important thing was the safe arrival of my babies and I was grateful to modern medicine for giving them to me. I thought in the 'old days' or in a Third World country we could have all died.

Louise: Finally the day came. My parents drove down from the country that morning. Tony, my step-son Eliot, Mum, Dad and I drove to the hospital to have two babies. We talked about what sex they'd be. We had eight names chosen. Four boys' names and four girls' names. I was expecting them both to be boys, my family always has boys. I had six nephews but no nieces. I prayed for a girl.

We waited in the hospital foyer with other people booked in for operations. One by one, patients and their families or friends were taken to their rooms. Finally our turn came. My room looked like an up-market motel. Comfy armchairs, floral curtains, television, phone, fridge. We sat around killing time. People came in occasionally to do things to me and tell me things. I hadn't eaten since the night before. Or was it that morning? Waiting, waiting. Even at this stage of my pregnancy I couldn't imagine two babies outside my body. In the weeks before I would put their rug on the floor and try to imagine two babies on it but always drew a blank. Maybe if you know the sex of your babies it's easier to imagine them. The sex of the babies was definitely the talking point that day. The woman who did our ultrasounds during the pregnancy asked if we wanted to know the sex. No way, thanks. 'You'll be really pleased,' she said. What did that mean? One of each, definitely. Or maybe two girls, maybe we'd said our family was full of boys? Then again, perhaps she meant we'd be really pleased regardless. A hint that wasn't a hint. I'm glad we left it until they were born.

Tony was coming into theatre with me. I was taken down in the lift in a wheelchair, dressed in a hospital gown. I filled in forms, was weighed and labelled for allergies. Still waiting. We were assigned a nurse. Sonya. I was put on a trolley and she held my hand and talked gently to me. Tony was taken away and dressed in theatre clothes. The operation before ours was running late. I was getting agitated waiting on a trolley in the hallway.

Suddenly it all happened so fast. We were in there. Tony was terrified, panicking, counting people. Talk to me, Tony. Calm me down. Where was Sonya? I needed her. I felt completely alone and terrified. I expected relaxing drugs but there were none, just the anaesthetist rubbing cold stuff on my back then injecting me with something to numb me from the arms down. I was petrified that he'd miss the spot and paralyse me. He hit the right spot, though and it numbed me but within about a minute I started to shake violently. 'Is this right? I'm shaking, I'm freezing, has something gone wrong? They've forgotten I'm here. Tony? Sonya? Someone?' Then the anaesthetist noticed me. It's OK, it's normal this happens to lots of people, it's just the anaesthetic. I was still shaking violently but I felt reassured. He was my man, the anaesthetist, he would look after me. Very selfish, I thought, to be preoccupied with myself as my babies were about to come into the world.

Two obstetricians, two paediatricians, two midwives, a few theatre nurses, some orderlies, Tony and my anaesthetist. Seventeen people. They put a green cloth up as a screen between the incision and me. I could feel him doing something, cutting or pulling, then suddenly they were saying, 'It's a girl.' Already? That was so quick. A girl, a girl, how wonderful, but that means the little one's a boy. They passed me a baby but she didn't look like mine. Was she the right one? She didn't look like she belonged to me. I held her on my chest for a minute or two. My baby. Then they pulled out my little one. He said, 'It's another girl.' Oh my God, two girls! My mum will be so happy. But they whisked her away. She wasn't breathing properly, needed resuscitation. My doctor, he insisted on a caesarean, he must have known something was wrong.

Tony was told to take photos but I knew he had a much more important job to do. I was yelling at him. 'Quick Tony, name the babies, which is which?' I needed to know who was who now. I had an overwhelmingly urgent need for them to be named immediately. Somehow it would establish their identity. One was Camille, the other Celeste, but Tony had to decide. He chose perfectly.

The babies were taken away before they'd finished repairing my caesar. Tony stayed with me until they wheeled me out of theatre then raced up to see his baby girls. I seemed to be in recovery forever. Everyone else was up with the babies. I couldn't stop talking to my nurse. Telling him about my girls, asking him questions. I missed them already and was desperate to get up there. He kept taking my blood pressure and watching me. I was so impatient to be upstairs, feeling alone, wanting to be with the girls. So impatient. Strange to be so alone and so separate from my baby girls; they were with everyone except me, after all we'd been through. Also strange that I had no partner with me after this frightening experience. It was one of those moments in life when I realised that we're ultimately alone. Finally they took me up.

Celeste, weighing in at 2.2 kg, had been put into a clear plastic box called an isolette to make sure her temperature remained constant. The orderlies wheeled me past her in the nursery to reassure me and let me know where she was. Camille, weighing 3.2 kg, must have been in my room with me but I honestly don't remember a thing from then on.

What a day.

Deciding how and when you will give birth

The most important thing about the birth of your twins is that you give birth as a healthy mother with two healthy babies. Your doctor may consider some or all of the following factors when judging the 'risk' involved in your pregnancy. The higher the risk is considered to be, the less choice you may have in relation to the birth. The following factors are relevant:

- how healthy you are
- your age
- the health of your babies
- the size of your babies
- whether you had fertility treatment
- whether you've previously had a baby
- the position of your babies in the uterus
- the position of the placenta(s)
- the number of amniotic sacs
- the resources available at your chosen hospital

Some women hope to deliver vaginally, others opt for a caesarean. Try to keep an open mind about the options and make a flexible plan.

Different hospitals have different policies and some have fairly strict policies on how they will handle twin births. Most hospitals automatically regard all twin pregnancies as high risk. Others have rules about monitoring the babies' progress and in what circumstances they will recommend a caesarean birth. They may also have rules about the number of obstetricians, paediatricians, midwives and support people who will be present. Some hospitals automatically use IV lines and epidurals for twin births, while others don't. If you have specific wishes about what you would and wouldn't like, let the staff know so they can fulfil them where possible.

Position of the babies in your uterus

Twin one is the baby presenting first (closest to the birth canal) in pregnancy, and is usually (but not always) born first whether vaginally or by caesarean. The most common position for twins in utero is heads down. This is also the best position for a vaginal birth. The first-born is often, but not always, bigger.

The next most common position is twin one with head down but twin two either feet down or crossways. Some obstetricians will insist on a caesarean birth for these twins.

Breech birth

In a breech birth, the baby's feet or bottom are nearest the cervix and are born first, followed by the largest part, which is the head. Breech birth is risky, even in a single pregnancy and particularly in a first pregnancy because the pelvis hasn't shown it can cope with a baby fitting through. If the head doesn't fit it's dangerous to find this out when the baby is already in the birth canal. It could result in trauma for both and possibly death of the baby.

Some obstetricians will deliver the first baby vaginally then deliver the second baby breech (feet first) vaginally. Sometimes the doctor puts his/her hand into the vagina to pull the second baby out by the foot.

Another option when twins are lying in this position is to give birth to the first baby vaginally then the second baby can be turned around to a head-down position for a vaginal birth too. You need to have already had an epidural in order for the second baby to be turned. Turning the second baby is done after the first twin is born. She is turned by pushing on the outside of your belly.

When twin one is not head-down it is a no-choice-caesarean. This is regardless of the position of your second baby. The reason that having the first baby born breech is so dangerous is that the two babies' chins can lock together and then both can get stuck in the birth canal.

- Fifty per cent of women carrying twins have a caesarean and this rate is steadily climbing.
- Most obstetricians and midwives like your second baby to be born less than 30 minutes after your first.

Who should be with you when you give birth?

You may be surprised by the number of medical staff at the birth of your babies. You may have a couple of surgeons, one or two anaesthetists, a couple of midwives, two paediatricians and some theatre nurses. You will probably want your partner or someone close to you, too. During a vaginal birth, the staff may change shifts. The presence of someone you know is comforting, even though they may feel a bit useless or in the way. Talk with your partner about what you are both expecting and how you imagine your support person is going to be helpful.

In theatre you might like to ask one midwife to stay with you and talk you through the birth. Hospitals generally let partners or a loved one into theatre too, unless you are having a general anaesthetic.

When should your babies be born?

Twins are healthier when they are born slightly earlier than 40 weeks. This is because the placenta loses its 'oomph' sooner in a twin pregnancy so doesn't function as well in those last couple of weeks. The optimum gestational age for twins is 35–38 weeks but if the babies' or mother's health is at risk the babies must come out, ready or not.

Pre-term labour

You will have already discussed with your doctor where you should go if you go into labour early. The number of weeks at which you can go to your chosen hospital will depend on the hospital's facilities. A pre-term birth in a large hospital with a Neonatal Intensive Care Unit (NICU) and a Special Care Nursery means you'll probably be close by your babies.

If you are in labour early and go to a smaller hospital, you may be transferred to a hospital with the facilities to look after all of you before the birth. If there's no time to transfer you, your babies may be transferred as soon as they're born to a larger hospital with specialised care for pre-term babies. Sometimes the babies can be sent to two different hospitals if there is a shortage of NICU beds. If you are too sick to move, or a bed isn't available, you may all spend some time separated. This can be stressful and worrying for you and your partner.

Chances are your babies won't come far too early, as only six per cent of twins are born pre-term. This is two and a half times the rate for a singleton pregnancy but is still not frequent. Most hospitals will admit babies born under 32 weeks into NICU, unless they are doing extremely well. If your babies are born at 32 weeks they will still be early but not generally dangerously early.

Just make sure you know the signs of pre-term labour (see page 50) so you can call your doctor or midwife or go straight to hospital as soon as you experience any of them.

Induced labour

If your labour is being induced, it means your doctor or midwife is preparing you for a vaginal birth. It means you haven't gone into labour naturally, so you will be given some help to get your contractions started. This may be done for your health, your babies' health or if your pregnancy has gone on too long.

There are a few different ways to start your labour:

- If your cervix hasn't begun to soften and hasn't dilated at all you could be given a hormone called prostaglandin. It is usually given in gels that are syringed into the cervix (at the back of your vagina). The gels are often given twice, one at night and one the next morning. This should start the cervix softening. The contractions may start within an hour or longer, or they may not start at all.

- If your cervix is already ripening (softening), and if the presenting twin's head has 'dropped', labour is sometimes induced by rupturing your membranes (breaking your waters). Your waters are broken with a device such as an 'amnihook', which looks like a knitting needle with a crotchet hook on the end. It's guided into the cervix during a vaginal examination and the hook is used to catch the membrane and tear a hole in it. If there are two amniotic sacs, the presenting one will be broken. Pain relief isn't usually given before this procedure, and it feels similar to a vaginal examination. This helps the contractions to commence.

- With a twin pregnancy, there often will have been some contractions so the cervix can already be ripe. Then you just need help to start the contractions. This is done by giving you a drug called oxytocin (brand name Syntocinon) through a continuous IV needle into your arm or the back of your hand. The pump slowly increases the amount given until your contractions are strong and steady. If the contractions come on too quickly the pump can be adjusted so they slow down. When it's started using oxytocin labour usually comes on harder and faster than it does with spontaneous labour. You don't have the benefit of getting used to the gradual increase in intensity of the contractions so it can seem more painful.

Some women just need some help getting started and find their contractions become strong, regular and continue on their own, so their oxytocin doses are stopped.

If labour hasn't begun after about six hours of oxytocin, a caesarean is usually the only option. The oxytocin doesn't affect the anaesthetics used for surgery.

Vaginal birth

If you and your doctor are planning a vaginal birth, look out for the following signs of labour:

- One baby's head drops into the pelvis, some women feel a greater heaviness or more pressure in their pelvis.
- You feel an intense burst of energy – try not to use it all up.
- You have a bloody 'show' which is a vaginal discharge that's clear, pink or brown mucus-blood. Your labour could begin between 24 and 48 hours later.
- An aching or cramping in your tummy and loose or frequent bowel movements and/or backache.
- When contractions begin at full term, many women with single babies stay home during the first stages of labour. With twins you usually contact your hospital as soon as your contractions are regular and about ten minutes apart and you're feeling like you have to breathe through them. A good indication is that you can't talk through them. Ring your doctor, midwife or the hospital if you're nervous or unsure about whether to go in.
- Your waters breaking. This can be a dribble or a gush. It means the amniotic sac has ruptured. Your babies may be coming, or it may be a sign of infection or it could be caused by the increasing pressure of your two babies. Check the colour of the amniotic fluid so you know if either of the babies have pooed (brown or green) and let your hospital know. If they've pooed, they'll be watched more closely for signs of distress during your labour, and when they are born, their mouths and throats will be suctioned thoroughly. They could also be taken to the nursery for oxygen monitoring. Some women carry maternity pads with them in case their waters break when they're out, and put a waterproof liner or towel under the bed sheet during the third trimester in case their waters break in bed.

During labour your pulse, blood pressure and breathing rate will be monitored at regular intervals. A midwife will probably examine you internally to check how far your cervix has dilated (how big the opening of your birth canal is). You may be asked to give a urine sample to check for sugar, protein and ketones. Your blood pressure will be monitored. Your urine will be checked regularly throughout your labour.

Most women having twins are given an intravenous line (IV) so they don't become dehydrated. The IV also helps prevent low blood pressure. Once it's hooked up, medication can also be given through the IV line.

Foetal monitor

A foetal monitor is a small clip-like device which may be attached to your presenting baby's head through the cervix so the heart rate can be monitored. The second baby may have their heart rate monitored on the outside of your belly. Whenever babies are induced, they are monitored for at least some period of time after you've been given oxytocin, or if your membranes have been ruptured. With twins, monitoring is often continued throughout labour using a machine called a cardiotocograph (CTG).

Your contractions will be monitored as well, using a gadget called a transducer connected to your tummy.

> (ANOTHER MUM SAYS) 'I hated the machine that measured my contractions. It meant my husband could sit and watch it and tell me how 'bad' or 'easy' my contractions were.'

Sometimes the position of the babies, cords, placentas and amount of fluid in the amniotic sac are measured using ultrasound during your labour. The ultrasound can be handy for the medical staff to see exactly what's going on and plan a course of action. Ultrasound can also be used to monitor progress if your second baby is being delivered breech or is being turned.

Forceps

Forceps resemble a pair of metal tongs that are inserted through the vagina to assist with the birth of the baby. Forceps called a 'lift out' are still used if the mother is very tired and it helps with the birth of the babies' heads. They are used during the final stages of delivery but are less likely to be used if your baby's head is still high in the cervix. A caesarean birth is often preferred over a difficult forceps birth.

Vacuum assisted birth

When a soft cup with a suction pump attached (called a ventouse) is placed on your baby's head, this is a vacuum assisted birth. The suction helps to move your baby down through the pelvis. It can often be used for the birth of your second twin if the cervix closes slightly after the birth of your first, as you don't need to be fully dilated for a ventouse delivery. There is debate about the risks of doctors without experience using this technique, so remember to discuss it with your doctor or midwife at a check-up rather than waiting until you are in labour.

Episiotomy

To make your vaginal opening wider or to prevent it tearing, a cut may be made in the perineum (the skin between your vagina and rectum). Perineal massage during pregnancy may make the area more easily stretched and help you to avoid an episiotomy. An episiotomy is done in 80–90 per cent of first vaginal births and 50 per cent of subsequent births. The cut is usually done as the baby's head begins to stretch the perineum. The decision about whether or not you need an episiotomy isn't made until the first baby's head crowns and the doctors can judge whether you look like you will tear. The main reasons for an episiotomy at this stage of the birth is that it can stop you tearing in a jagged, hard-to-repair way, and that it can also cut down pushing time by up to 30 minutes. It's often done if your baby gets distressed and needs to be delivered quickly.

Urinary catheter

If you have an epidural, you will probably have a urinary catheter. The catheter is basically a long, thin tube inserted into your urethra in order to empty your bladder contents into a bag. A full bladder can be damaged by the babies during the birth or may slow down their progress through the birth canal. The epidural also means you'll have numbness in your bottom half, so you won't be able to tell when you need to pee and you may lose muscle control. You may feel like you're doing a poo when you're not, but if you do, don't worry.

First stage of labour

This lasts from your first regular contractions through to when your cervix is fully dilated at 10 cm. This stage is often a couple of hours shorter for those having twins than for those having one baby. The cervix of women pregnant with twins tends to dilate (open up) more quickly.

This first stage has three parts: early labour, active labour and transitional labour.

Early labour is where you may be up to 4 cm dilated and might feel excited and talkative and possibly hungry. The contractions might feel manageable. You will probably be allowed to suck ice but not eat and drink because of the chance of needing an emergency caesarean. For a twin and a first pregnancy this stage usually lasts 6–8 hours, with the contractions being irregular and lasting around 30–45 seconds each.

Active labour lasts about 3–4 hours. Contractions are stronger, lasting 45–60 seconds. An epidural may be started during active labour. If your waters haven't broken, your doctor or midwife might decide to break them, as it speeds up the labour and the colour of the amniotic fluid can be checked and an internal foetal monitor put on your presenting baby's head so the heart rate can be watched more closely. If they break your waters, you might hear a pop, then feel a gush of fluid coming from your vagina. Sometimes contractions stop at this point as the uterus has lost tone. You may be given oxytocin through your IV line to start contractions again.

If the baby being delivered is facing forwards instead of towards your back, you can get severe pain from the head pressing on the nerves in your lower back and the pressure on the last bone in your spine (coccyx). Staying off your back, leaning forward and rocking can help.

Transitional labour is your opportunity to swear and scream at your partner (if you haven't done so already). Using your voice can make you feel stronger and making whatever noise you feel like is usually encouraged. The transitional stage ought only to last about an hour. The contractions are very intense, lasting 60–90 seconds and coming every three minutes. You might vomit or feel nauseous or have hot or cold flushes or the shakes. Ask for blankets to warm you up and comfort you.

During this transitional time you may have an incredible urge to push.

You will be guided by your doctor or obstetrician and if it's not time to push, you'll be encouraged to pant or blow with your contractions until your cervix is completely dilated. If you push before you are fully dilated, it can damage your cervix or cause it to become swollen. The swelling could slow the birth.

Second stage of labour

This involves pushing and the birth of your two babies. It is usually longer with twins than with one baby because there are two babies to come out. If it's your first vaginal delivery this stage usually takes 1–2 hours, with the second baby coming between 15 and 30 minutes after the first. It is likely to be quicker if you've previously had a vaginal birth.

During this stage you may feel you have more control because you can push. If you've had an epidural, you may not feel completely numb. With modern 'cocktail' epidurals you often feel sensations without the pain. You may still be able to walk and feel when you should push without feeling abdominal pain. You don't have to lie on your back, and staying upright lets gravity help you along. As the contractions are happening, try to see in your mind your baby moving down that birth canal as you push.

You may be given a mirror on a stand as your baby crowns, when you can actually see your baby's head starting to come through the vaginal opening, to watch the head appear then turn as the shoulders come through. The rest of your first baby then slips out.

The first baby's umbilical cord will be clamped in two places, then cut. He or she may be wrapped and placed on your tummy and may have a warm hat popped on her head to stop her losing heat or the neonatal team will take over your first baby straightaway, possibly give her some oxygen and maybe suction her through the mouth. This gets rid of any mucous, amniotic fluid, secretions or meconium that could cause her to have lung problems. The oxygen is given if your baby is distressed or is slow to cry. She'll probably have an identification band put on one wrist and maybe on one ankle.

Meanwhile, you will be giving birth to your second baby. This baby will now have room to move and if necessary room to be turned and a foetal heart monitor attached to his or her head. When the baby gets into the head-down position, you can begin pushing again to give birth vaginally.

If the birth slows down for the second baby, things may be hurried along by:

- injecting oxytocin to bring back contractions, or
- breaking the waters of the second baby, or
- a 'helping hand' from your doctor or obstetrician.

If the second baby is in a breech position the doctor may use forceps to help him or her through the birth canal. For both of these types of breech delivery and for turning a baby an epidural is used – as well as numbing the pain, it relaxes the uterus and makes using forceps or the doctor's hand more comfortable for you.

Third stage of labour

In this stage the placenta(s) are delivered. Within two minutes of the birth the placenta(s) begin to separate from the wall of the uterus. The doctor checks them thoroughly to make sure none has been left inside. Retained bits can cause haemorrhage or infection. If a lot of placenta has been left inside the uterus you may need to go to theatre for it to be removed surgically. If the placenta has come away well but your per-ineum has torn, or if you had an episiotomy, you will probably be stitched up at this point.

ANOTHER MUM SAYS   'I was induced at 38 weeks when I was just too tired, swollen and uncomfortable. It was funny to be driving to hospital calmly and not actually in labour. I had never imagined it that way. I'd previously asked the obstetrician if I could be fitted with the epidural line without the drugs initially. I wanted it to be in place just in case while also giving myself the opportunity to go it alone and experience childbirth. The epidural line was fitted before I even had a contraction and I'm really glad I had it. My waters were broken at 11.30 a.m. and I was given Syntocinon and a catheter was inserted. For a few hours I didn't feel much, then wham the contractions came full on and close together. The pain was huge and I went deep inside myself. I rocked my body on the spot, it was hard to move around. After about seven hours I was nearly fully dilated and feeling the urge to push. Somehow I had the presence of mind to ask for the pain relief then, as I knew it needed to be in place before the second one was due, in case the baby needed to be 'fished out' by the doctor. Once the pain was gone I 'came back' into the room and could talk again.

I pushed out my first baby at 8.40 p.m. and the doctor assisted with forceps. I couldn't feel a thing and was very grateful for the epidural. I pushed him out and Baby One was placed on my tummy and looked up at me contentedly. My belly quickly deflated and the doctor broke the waters of the second baby which had started to move around. The doctor went in 'elbow up' and was fishing around for a limb. This was difficult to do and took a long time. The hardest work I've ever done is delivering my second baby. He was coming out leg first. After nearly 30 minutes the midwife said, 'You're going to have to get this baby out now' and I could sense the urgency in her voice. At that point my husband said 'It's a boy' and those two comments gave me the motivation I needed to dig deep inside myself to find the energy to push him out. Baby Two was placed next to me and was grunting but looking very sluggish and confused. He was taken straight to the trolley for the second twin which had lots more medical stuff at the ready. There was no movement in his limbs and all we could see was a huge mask over his head and his chest humping up and down with each breath.

I was having placentas pulled out of me but was very focused on my baby and eager to know if he was all right. Mind you, as the placentas were being dragged out of me they made a huge farting noise and I turned to the obstetrician and said, 'Oh, excuse me.' Funny in times of amazing stress and uncertainty one should be so polite. Baby Two was taken to the Special Care Nursery but he was OK – he needed to be kept warm and monitored for a while.'

Caesarean birth

(ANOTHER MUM SAYS) 'I didn't have a contraction.'

About half of all sets of twins are born using a caesarean section. This is surgery with the babies taken out through a cut about 12–15 cm long through your belly and uterus at the bikini line. The babies are pulled out through this cut. Sometimes you know in advance that you will be having a caesarean. The reason(s) for a planned caesarean include the following situations:

- Your presenting twin is in a breech position.
- You have small babies who may find labour too stressful.
- Your twins are in the same amniotic sac and their umbilical cords risk being tangled during a vaginal delivery.
- You had complications during a previous vaginal birth.
- You haven't had a previous vaginal birth. Some doctors believe the labour in this case could be too long and stressful for the second baby.
- One or both your babies has congenital defects where it's potentially dangerous to deliver vaginally.
- Conjoined twins are always delivered using a caesarean.
- You have genital herpes. Don't assume if you see or feel no sores it is safe to deliver vaginally. Get your doctor or midwife to check for internal sores too.
- You choose to have a caesarean.
- Your obstetrician advises a caesarean.

Planned caesarean

Your doctor will discuss a date to book you in to the hospital, usually around 36–38 weeks gestation. This assumes you won't go into labour before this date. Admission to hospital for a planned caesarean usually involves filling in paperwork, having your vital signs checked and blood taken by midwives. You'll have to sign a consent form for surgery and the anaesthetic. All of this may happen in your room or ward.

Nail polish, jewellery and dentures are usually removed. An IV (intra-venous) line is usually started in your arm or the back of your hand. This can be done in your room or ward or when you're taken in to surgery. The top of your pubic area will probably be shaved. This keeps the area where the cut is made clean and so that the sticky bandages don't pull hairs when removed. Your pubic hair grows back over the scar so you'll only see it when you have a Brazilian XXX bikini wax.

You'll probably then be wheeled to surgery where your belly can be cleaned with antiseptic. A catheter is usually inserted to keep your bladder empty. Once you've arrived in theatre you'll be given either an epidural or spinal block so you can stay awake for the birth of your babies. You may feel pressure and pulling during the operation but no pain and you'll be fully alert for the birth of your babies.

You can choose to have a general anaesthetic for a caesarean – staying awake is the mother's choice, not something that you have to do.

Emergency caesareans

When your health or the health of your babies is threatened, an emergency caesarean may be carried out. The reason could be any of the following:

- One or both babies are severely distressed and need to come out quickly.
- There is bleeding signifying possible placental abruption (placenta is coming off the wall of the uterus) or a tear in the umbilical cord.
- The mother has eclampsia which can cause a stroke.
- The umbilical cord comes out before the baby (cord prolapse), potentially blocking the baby's oxygen and blood supply.

With an emergency caesarean, depending on the circumstances, you may be given an epidural or a spinal block (numbing from the breasts down while you stay awake) or a general anaesthetic (making you completely unconscious). Regardless of which method is used, it's unlikely that you'll feel any pain. The anaesthetist is there so if you feel anything at all let them know.

In the operating theatre

Partners are allowed in the operating theatre for a caesarean, although not usually if it involves a general anaesthetic. Your partner wears a surgical suit and sits close to your head so you can talk throughout the operation. Your blood pressure will be monitored using a blood pressure cuff, and there'll be a clip attached to one of your fingers to measure your oxygen levels. A screen is put up blocking your view of your belly so you can't see the operation.

The cut through your skin is made quite low, just below where your pubic hair grows. Then another side-to-side cut is made through your uterus. This type of incision means it's possible to have a vaginal delivery with your next pregnancy without risk of rupturing the scar. If your babies are very pre-term, you may have to have a longer vertical cut because the uterus mightn't be developed enough to use a side-to-side cut.

You shouldn't feel pain during the operation but you may feel tugging and pulling so you may feel suddenly sick. Dizziness and nausea can be caused by a drop in blood pressure. If you do feel sick tell the anaesthetist who may give you medication through your IV to stop the nausea. You may be given extra fluids.

From the start of the actual surgery to the time your first baby is born takes about five minutes. Your second baby will be born within another few minutes. Each of their umbilical cords is cut and the babies might be passed to you one-by-one for a quick hold. Then they'll probably be dried, warmed, evaluated and given oxygen or suction.

Your doctor then removes the placentas making sure there are no bits left inside. They often lift the uterus out to check for signs of bleeding, then the uterus, muscles and skin are sewn back together. The outside skin is either stapled or stitched. All of this mending takes about 45 minutes.

First twin vaginal, second twin caesarean

It does happen, but thankfully very rarely (in less than one per cent of twin deliveries). No doctor would plan to put you through this but sometimes the second delivery becomes an emergency. It may happen if the second baby becomes distressed. The first sign of distress is usually a change to the baby's heart rate, generally with it slowing down but not returning quickly back to normal. An emergency caesarean may also be needed for birth of the second baby if the placenta starts breaking away from the wall of the uterus or if the second baby's cord falls down through the cervix, threatening to block the oxygen supply.

Obviously this is an extremely exhausting way to deliver twins. Stay as long as you can in hospital to recover your strength. You will need to follow the usual steps to recover from surgery – you will have had an operation, as well as giving birth to two babies.

Pain relief

Epidural anaesthetic

Epidurals are often recommended for the birth of twins because of the increased chances of a caesarean. If it becomes necessary, the doctors can move quickly to a caesarean without having to give you a general anaesthetic. It also has a relaxing effect on your uterus so during a vaginal delivery it can make it easier if necessary for your doctor to turn your baby or deliver him or her breech.

The anaesthetist cleans your lower back with an antiseptic solution then injects a numbing solution into your skin. This numbs the area where a larger needle is put in, and a tiny little catheter tube is poked down through that needle into the space between your bones and spinal cord. This area is called the epidural space. This is a highly skilled action, which can be considered dangerous because of potential damage to the spinal cord if the needle goes too far. The catheter can be left in without being used, so that it's in place if you decide you want pain relief or need an emergency caesarean. When you are given the drug, you'll probably feel the full numbness in about 15 minutes. It's a heavy feeling and your legs feel clumsy. Less epidural is used for a vaginal birth than a caesarean. With a vaginal birth, you'll still feel and should be able to move, and you may have pins and needles. For a caesarean you will be numb from the breasts down with no movement. The anaesthetist tailors the amount of anaesthetic you need, completely blocking any pain. An epidural can cause your blood pressure to drop but the theatre staff will be keeping a close eye on you. Another common complaint is a 'spinal headache'. This is a severe headache that comes on after your delivery and is caused by your spinal fluid level dropping. Lying flat may help and if it doesn't, ask for pain relief.

Spinal block

A spinal block is usually used with forceps or caesarean births but can be given for a vaginal birth. It is an analgesic fluid injected into the spinal fluid in the spinal canal. The lower part of your body starts to go numb immediately and you can't move your legs. This lack of feeling lasts for a couple of hours. Spinal blocks can cause your blood pressure to drop so you may need extra fluids through your IV line. There is also an inability to urinate, a need to lie flat for 6–12 hours after the block and a possible headache.

Spinal/epidural combination

This is a combination of the spinal block analgesic and the epidural anaesthetic. It also provides rapid pain relief then ongoing numbness. This combination may be used late in labour when instant pain relief is needed. The spinal block lasts about one hour while it takes about half an hour for the longer lasting epidural to kick in.

General anaesthetic

A general anaesthetic is given in an emergency or if an epidural has failed, or in a planned caesarean if the mother chooses to have one. The anaesthetic is given through an IV and the mother is put to sleep for the birth. It can have an anaesthetic affect on the babies. If the babies stop breathing or their heart rates slow right down from the anaesthetic, they may be given Narcan to reverse this effect.

> (ANOTHER MUM SAYS) 'With me being asleep during the caesarean, my husband was able to get some great video of everything I missed. I watched it all later with great delight. Coming out of the anaesthetic was distressing, I was very disoriented and demanded to know where my babies were. My husband was also confused and distressed after the birth, torn between staying with me in recovery and going with the girls to the nursery.'

Nitrous oxide

This gas is mixed with oxygen and given to you through a mask that you hold and so control the amount you receive. It provides pain relief without interfering with your contractions. It can help with 'breathing through' contractions, making it easier to relax. Gas causes some women to have funny thoughts or even to hallucinate while they're using it.

Pethidine

This pain-killer can be given in early labour to help you relax, or in the extremely painful transitional period. It is administered via a quick stab of a needle in the thigh. Pethidine only works for a couple of hours and sometimes doesn't actually help with the pain but relaxes you. It does have side effects which can include a drop in blood pressure, vomiting and respiratory depression. It can also slow your labour down because it relaxes your uterus. Pethidine is usually avoided in the final hour before babies are born because it can have an effect on their breathing and heart rate. As with a general anaesthetic, the babies may need Narcan to counter the effects of pethidine.

Alternative methods of pain relief

There are alternative pain management methods that may be worth discussing in antenatal classes or with your midwife or physiotherapist. These include use of breathing techniques, massage, hypnotherapy and music.

TIPS FOR SURVIVING BIRTH

- Have a birth plan. You will have a choice within reason and as long as you and your babies are doing well.
- Keep an open mind, be prepared for any contingency or complication.
- Think about who you'd like to support you through the birth.
- Plan what you want your support person to do if the babies go to the special care nursery. Will they go with them or stay with you? You don't have to stick to the plan on the day but you'll be prepared in case this happens.
- Ask the midwives whenever you're not sure about what's happening.
- Speak up. If you want privacy, music, whatever you want, the staff will probably do their best to provide it.
- Have as much pain relief as you want during the birth and in the following days.

TIPS FOR PARTNERS

- Know which hospital to head for if your babies come early. And know how to get there.
- Know what to expect from a vaginal birth and from a caesarean birth, read about them and ask friends who have been through it.
- Even if you're feeling frightened or unsure, don't forget your partner – support and encourage her.
- Make sure you have the list of phone numbers to start ringing around with the good news.
- Hold her hand if she wants you to and pull your head in when she tells you to.

Why are you crying?

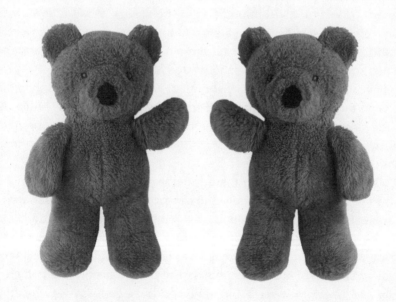

HOSPITAL

HOSPITAL: OUR STORIES

Katrina: I was woken some time on the Sunday night that my girls were born, so that I could feed them. I actually felt very annoyed. I just needed to sleep and there we were trying to establish a complicated feeding ritual. I had no idea what time it was and was lying prostrate and helpless on the bed – the whole experience seemed so surreal.

The midwives were very experienced and just grabbed my nipples and squashed them into tiny newborn mouths. The midwives stayed and held the babies during this process then whisked them back to the Special Care Nursery.

I had decided that I wanted to master feeding one baby at a time first and then aim for twin feeding. I'm glad I didn't bother with this. Learning to twin feed was more important. I could always master one at a time later, if necessary.

That first day when I tried to get out of bed for the shower and loo, I fainted. I'd lost too much blood and my iron levels were too low. I was given a choice between having a blood transfusion, or eating liver every day and staying in bed for the next three months. Both the liver and the bed rest sounded impossible, so four bags of blood it was.

Initially the girls' nappies were changed by the midwives and then the girls were brought to my room for feeds every three and a half hours. At first they weren't getting quite enough breastmilk from me so the midwives gave them some supplementary feeds through the tubes in their noses during that first week.

It was very difficult feeding them together comfortably on the single, narrow hospital bed. I had to have the cage sides up and pillows strategically placed so as not to lose a baby down the side. I always needed help from one of the midwives to get it all set up. They couldn't always rush to my side when I buzzed. Sometimes I was lying almost helpless while my babies screamed for milk. I kept thinking, 'If there was only one baby …'

Ella and Charlotte were a bit jaundiced but otherwise very healthy. They were in the Special Care Nursery mainly because they were a month early and only weighed two kilos each. The paediatrician wanted a close professional eye kept on them. Midwives monitored the girls' temperatures, nappies and growth.

The blood transfusion pepped me up so my babies were moved into my room. I was desperate to have them with me, but also terrified about being responsible for them. That first night was an absolute disaster. The building's airconditioning was out of whack and despite being firmly wrapped in blankets and beanies my babies were freezing and cried all night. None of us slept. I could barely get out of bed, and I didn't feel capable of snuggling two babies in my single hospital bed all night. The paediatrician was very cross that their temperatures had dropped overnight in my room and insisted they be put back in the Special Care Nursery. I worried about the girls not being with me even though I knew they were in the best hands.

By this time I was a wreck and wasn't able to think rationally. The midwives put the 'No Visitors' sign up, intercepted people, and took phone messages from the desk. Only close family and my best friend were allowed in. There were literally only about four other visitors I saw during my hospital stay. I had to focus on myself, my husband and our girls. As a result I have learnt not to ring or visit new mums while they're still in hospital, unless asked!

My nipples were cracking and bleeding, making feeding very uncomfortable. A kind midwife encouraged me to express milk for a while to give my nipples a rest. So at 3 a.m. Thursday morning I was mastering the hospital pump and doing a crash course in bottles and sterilisation. It was a huge relief and gave my nipples a chance to recover. After a day and a half the babies were reattached. From then on the breastfeeding was fine. While their initial attachment was toe-curlingly painful, once on, we were right.

Midwives came numerous times a day to check my incision, temperature, blood pressure and blood loss. They also delivered the paracetamol and liked to ask if I'd done a poo yet. Everyone got a good look at my breasts, from the cleaner, the food deliverer, the midwives, the paediatrician, my obstetrician, orthopedic surgeons and physios, all with their various assistants and the lovely but numerous church ladies who popped in with knitted coathangers – they all got an eyeful. I was usually topless, either feeding the babies or airing my nipples.

At birth Ella and Charlotte were diagnosed as having hip dysplasia (displaced hips). This is not an uncommon condition and it seems we met all the criteria that increase likelihood. That is, multiple birth, girls, breech birth (they were pulled out by their legs and bottoms), and Welsh descent! One symptom of this was Ella's leg being up over her head and her crooked knee, which was fixed with a splint. Her case appeared more severe, but ultrasounds showed Charlotte had the same condition. Ninety-five per cent of cases are fixed by wearing a Pavlic harness. The harness looks like Austrian lederhosen made with velcro and buckles. It went over and around each baby's body and legs to spread their legs, and raise their knees up to hip height. This was to help the girls' hip sockets form properly. If the harness treatment didn't work then an operation would be a possibility. Along with the harness, the treatment included wearing double nappies. This was to give extra bulk and weight to help keep the girls' legs spread and hips in place.

They couldn't wear normal baby clothes. They were in nighties all the time, socks over the top of the harness feet to keep their toes warm and big jumpers or cardigans. With their legs spread so wide, they only just squeezed into their baby capsules for the car.

In hospital I rode an emotional roller-coaster. I cried nearly all week, often with joy. I was thrilled with my girls and amazed by their beauty. I thought I was so clever. I was also delirious. I told my husband we could have another if he wanted a son! There were lots of times when I also felt sorry for myself and for my babies. I doubted my ability to look after them both. I felt we would all be better off if they'd come three years apart. I wasn't used to needing help, and I resented asking for it, and not being able to manage without it. If there was only one baby I would be managing fine, I kept telling myself, the anger building up inside.

Sometimes I preferred one baby to the other. I know this sounds terrible, but I'd look at one baby and say that was the one I didn't want. It took a while for me to realise that even if sometimes one baby was more demanding than the other – and they did take turns in this – that I still loved them both. These feelings were very much part of my coming to terms with their being two.

By the end of our first week in hospital, I was a new woman. I loved having my body back and being able to sleep comfortably. I enjoyed being hungry again and eating all the time. I was able to sit up comfortably, walk around, shower and just feel happy. The girls were pretty much confined to the Special Care Nursery but they were allowed in my room for brief visits. We learnt we could have a 'pass out' and Brad and I took off for lunch in town, while the babies stayed in good hands in the Special Care Nursery.

Brad's work was very flexible and he was able to spend time in hospital with me each day. He was working from home and arranged his schedule so he could focus on the girls and me. He was able to bond with the girls and was an active father right from the start.

I was very anxious about having the staples from my caesarean removed, but it ended up being a simple procedure that felt like a hair being plucked.

We ended up staying in hospital for two weeks. I contracted some sort of virus at the end of the first week and had a 40-degree temperature with cold and hot fevers. The doctors were unable to determine the cause of my illness so I was being tested in every which way. I had X-rays, an ECG, a Pap smear, more blood tests. I think there was some concern that it was a side effect of surgery, but we still don't know.

I confided in a nurse how terrified I was at the thought of taking the girls home and being on my own with them and he arranged for the hospital social worker to come and see me. I told her how scared I was, but that I also thought it would be insane not to be scared, so that really I felt this was normal. She agreed, and gave me contact numbers so that when I got home, I knew how to get help should I need it.

The girls were making steady weight gains and spent our last night in hospital in the room with me and we all managed fine. They already had their dummies. I wasn't able to cuddle two babies as much as we all would have liked. I had thoughts that I couldn't just cuddle one, it wouldn't be fair to the other. I felt it had to be both or none. The dummy seemed to comfort them and if they were happy, so was I.

In the end I was desperate to get home and start my new life. I wanted to cuddle up to my husband in bed and my mum had arrived and was staying for the first six weeks to help us through.

Louise: For the first couple of days there were plenty of drugs supplied to stop the pain from my caesarean. I was given a green liquid in a cup that I think was morphine and some Voltaren suppositories that felt brilliant. I was disappointed to find I wasn't allowed to have any more suppositories after the first two days, their pain relief was extraordinary. Pulling myself up out of bed was agony at first but the nurses kept stressing how important it was to move around as much as possible and stop it hurting for longer. Walking was unbearable the first few times I got out of bed but then I came good quite quickly. It was tempting to stoop over and shuffle but I bit my lip and straightened out, imagining that if I didn't stand tall then I'd stiffen up for ever.

I had terrible stomach cramps for a couple of days after the operation. They were wind pains and are apparently quite common after giving birth. The nurses gave me warm peppermint water to sip. Once I'd done a poo and had no more wind, there was no more cramping.

My greatest worry before the girls were born was how I was going to handle visitors in the hospital and during the early days at home. I knew I'd get wound up and think too much about keeping visitors happy and entertained and not get used to my babies. We all had a big adjustment ahead. I knew I wanted to see very few people while in the hospital but did nothing to stop people coming. In fact I probably encouraged them.

I knew there would be a lot of interest in the girls while we were in hospital since people love seeing twins. They're special and fascinating. When they're newborn it's difficult to believe they both come from the same place. We had nine visitors on their first night in the world. From then on it didn't stop. The hospital only let people in during visiting hours but during those hours I had far too many. I wanted to see everyone while at the same time I knew I needed to spend quiet time with my new small family.

After a day or two Celeste was brought to my room for feeding but taken back to her warm little plastic box in between feeds. The first time she was brought to me she was wearing a green-and-white-striped beanie that was too big and looked silly. I thought the midwives were having a joke. Much later I realised they weren't being funny but were keeping her warm.

I kept Celeste with Camille and me as long as I could and the nurses would let her stay out longer and longer each day. I refused to think about her alone in her box, it was too upsetting and there was nothing I could do to change things. I kept telling myself everything would be all right, she'd be allowed out permanently soon. Already this was a situation where I couldn't protect her. She was so small and alone.

Camille stayed in my room in my bed. I was hanging on tight to forget about Celeste, distracting myself with Camille's comfort. I remember feeling as if I was somehow depending on her and this was a reversal of how things should be.

Overnight I fed the girls on a chair near the nursery. They were having a breastfeed and a formula feed from a bottle as well. I met and talked with a lot of other women feeding in the nursery overnight. My girls were latching on quite well but through my hospital stay and beyond, they continued to need the formula as well.

One morning I woke to find that someone had given them dummies overnight. It was odd that no one had asked me but it seemed that if I hadn't wanted them to have dummies I should've left a note in their cribs saying 'No dummies please'. So they got their dummies then and they weren't letting them go.

Once Celeste was out of her little warm box, I spent the time between feeding and visitors lying on the bed with her and Camille. They'd go to sleep and I'd pop them in their two little hospital cribs until they woke again. If one was awake while the other was still in her crib, I'd have this intense feeling of guilt. I felt sure I loved the one who was awake so much more than the other. She was so special, the other could never compete. Then, of course, they'd swap. The other baby would wake and she'd be the one I loved the most. This zig-zagging went on for at least the first year of their lives.

On the third day of the girls' life, I was a weepy mess. I was *sooo* happy and simultaneously *sooo* sad. It's joked about as 'third-day baby blues' but I thought I had quite a few things to take seriously. I had lived through IVF and as a result a nervous pregnancy. I'd stopped work, we didn't have much money, I'd had major abdominal surgery and biggest of all there were these two precious dependent babies. Oh my God . . . I felt an enormous combination of relief and trepidation. The last thing I needed was to feel obliged to be friendly and cheerful for anyone who wandered in.

After a couple of days, during the routine blood pressure checks the nurses went into a spin and it was decided that my blood pressure was going too high too fast and needed to be brought down quickly. I was given a drug that brought it down fast but gave me an immediate migraine that lasted for days. I was moved to a quiet room at the back of the hospital, away from the noisy nurses' station so I could get some peace and some sleep.

While I was sick, the girls stayed in the nursery except when they were feeding. With help from pain-killers I just slept and slept. Whenever I woke, I couldn't stand or walk because of the dizzy, unbalancing effects of the blood pressure drugs. I must have had a lot of help from those nurses to keep functioning.

My stay in hospital was expected to be about a week but because of the migraine and my high blood pressure it ended up being two. For the second week I put a sign on my door saying 'No visitors allowed – see nursing staff'. They were great at explaining to anyone who popped in that I wasn't up to it. I kept it there well after the migraine had vanished and savoured every undisturbed moment.

When the day came for us to leave the hospital I felt completely ready.

Recovery

Your obstetrician or the hospital's obstetrician will probably visit you regularly while you are in hospital to check on your recovery. They are looking after you, while paediatricians look after the babies. This is an opportunity to ask about the birth, if there's anything you can't remember or if you have any concerns or questions.

Hopefully the midwives will be in your room about six times a day, more often if you need help. When you think you may need help, pressing the buzzer straightaway will put you in the queue during those busy times. For all sorts of reasons, help isn't always available as quickly as you'd like.

The midwives' observations will probably include checking your blood pressure, taking your temperature and monitoring your blood loss by checking your sanitary pads. They may feel your tummy to check the size of your uterus to make sure it's hardening and shrinking. If you had stitches in your perineum, they will probably check those to make sure everything is healing as it should be and that there's no sign of infection. They will also probably check or ask about your breasts to make sure your nipples aren't getting sore and that there's no engorgement.

Regardless of the type of birth you had, there is a risk of deep vein thrombosis so your calves will probably also be checked. To avoid developing deep vein thrombosis it's important to keep active and exercise your legs. Even if you're in bed, you can bend your feet back and forth and stretch your calf muscles.

During pregnancy the physical and hormonal changes can affect your bowels, so midwives are often keen to ensure that's all working properly. Going to the toilet is often scary if you have stitches in your perineum or if your haemorrhoids are worse after the birth. They may also ask if you're peeing OK.

Bleeding

In the first few hours after the birth you'll be watched closely for signs of haemorrhage. As the stretched uterus shrinks back down it clamps the blood vessels in the muscles of the uterus and stops the bleeding. Because of the incredible stretching of the uterus in a twin pregnancy it is not uncommon to haemorrhage.

You may pass large clots of blood straight after the birth. These can be from where the placentas detached from the wall of the uterus and left wounds, or from any placenta or membranes left in the uterus. If you fill more than two sanitary pads in an hour or you pass a blood clot bigger than a 50 cent piece, you should notify a nurse straightaway. These clots will be checked for any sign of membrane or placenta. Retained placenta or membranes can stop the uterus from contracting and can also cause infection. If you have a smelly discharge, fever or pain, you may have an infection in the lining of your uterus that will need to be treated immediately with antibiotics. It can make you quite sick if it's not treated.

For some days after the birth you may pass more blood than if you'd had one baby. You need to wear long, large sanitary pads and have plenty of spare knickers on hand. Using tampons increases the risk of infection so it is discouraged.

The bleeding usually slows and turns from red to darker then a whitish yellow. The process may take up to six weeks. This is healthy and normal.

Pain relief

Staff will probably offer you relief if you're experiencing pain. Remember that if you are in pain, there is no need to suffer. Taking pain relief before you need it badly means you may be able to move around more easily, and you need to move in order to get better quickly. If you stiffen up, it makes moving much harder, and if you let the pain get on top of you, it can be much harder to get back in control.

An epidural or spinal anaesthetic usually fades after a few hours and has completely gone by about six hours. Some hospitals leave the epidural catheter in and give you top-ups for 24–48 hours, to give pain relief without making you numb. Narcotics are often given through IV, injection or suppositories initially. After a general anaesthetic you may be given a morphine PCA (patient controlled analgesia) or you may be given pethidine injections for 24–48 hours. After about 48 hours other analgesics given in tablet form usually do the trick. Be careful of those with codeine, which can cause constipation.

Patient controlled analgesia (PCA) is becoming quite common. The pain-killer is in a slow-infusion drip into the back of your hand and you can push a button to give yourself an extra dose. You can't overdose as the system won't let you have too much.

Feeling sick, sore and exhausted

You will probably experience some discomfort for the first few days after the birth of your twins. Your discomfort might include:

- Bleeding – mothers of twins can bleed more heavily after birth because of the extra stretching of the uterus, and because the placenta covered more of it.
- Cramping as your uterus contracts, sometimes called 'after pains' – your uterus has a lot of shrinking to do. This cramping can be more severe when you're breastfeeding because the hormone oxytocin, released during breastfeeding, causes these contractions. This means breastfeeding helps your uterus to shrink back into shape more quickly. For a while, some women find it helps to take paracetamol prior to feeding.
- Wind cramps or constipation – can be caused by anaesthetic and be really painful. Drink lots of water and sip peppermint water. Avoid fizzy drinks.
- Getting in and out of bed can be agony – roll off the bed, slowly and carefully, taking your time.
- If you've had stitches following a vaginal delivery or the delivery involved forceps you could be sore – salt baths can hasten healing, or push your tush under the warm tap.
- Legs can be sore or stiff, especially if they were in stirrups for the birth or for stitches. And all that pushing uses muscles you've never used before.
- A caesarean is major surgery and bits got tugged around in there that can take a while to resettle.
- Sore breasts and nipples – wearing a maternity bra all the time can help. For tips on breast and nipple care, see pages 154–155.
- Exhaustion – sleep and rest as much as possible. The demands of a twin pregnancy and the heavier bleeding can increase the likelihood of anaemia. Eating an iron-rich diet after as well as during your pregnancy will help.
- You may also urinate and sweat more than usual while your body expels some of the extra fluid stored during your pregnancy.

After a caesarean it's best to get up and walk as soon as possible to prevent deep vein thrombosis. The first time is painful. Try to time it after you've taken pain-killers so it won't be as bad. Take it slowly, you may need help.

It gets easier every time you stand up. Gentle and regular exercise, like walking up the corridor or stretching your legs and ankles in bed, helps everything, including your perineum, to return to normal more quickly.

If you don't have any energy or are unwell, ask the nurses or your partner to latch the babies on to your breasts or to express your milk for you with a breast pump.

It is possible to develop a urinary tract infection after all the pushing of a vaginal birth or after having had a catheter inserted into your bladder. Drinking two litres of water a day helps to prevent these urinary tract infections, and to avoid constipation. The water will dilute your urine so it won't sting as much if you have stitches or grazes around your perineum. If you can only do tiny amounts of urine or if it's dark, burning or smelly, let the nurses know, as you may have an infection. Another sign of infection is a high temperature.

Sore breasts

Your milk usually comes in during the first week and fills your breasts, making them look and feel full and heavy. You may be breastfeeding each baby eight or more times each day.

It is possible for your breasts to become so full that they are engorged, uncomfortable and hard and the babies can't drink. Hand-expressing breastmilk helps, as does massaging your breasts under a hot shower or applying a warm or cold pack. You can get immediate and excellent relief from a cold pack made by putting wet cloths in the freezer over a cup. They come out frozen and breast-shaped.

If you are not going to breastfeed or express, giving your breasts as little stimulation as possible stops them producing milk. There is a drug available to discourage your breasts from producing milk. Wearing a well-fitting bra and putting cold packs on your breasts will help.

For more information on blocked ducts and breast infections, see page 155.

Jelly belly

ANOTHER MUM SAYS 'I was chatting with some ladies at the hospital canteen and they asked me when my baby was due. I'd given birth two days ago. They were all smaller than me but still waiting to deliver.'

You will undoubtedly leave hospital smaller than when you went in – just like a health farm! However you mightn't be as small as you'd imagined. You may still be wearing your maternity clothes when you leave, or elastic or loose pants. Dress for comfort and give your body time. Your growth in pregnancy took many months, so allow it some months to return to 'normal'.

If you're used to firm abs, it may be a shock when you have a wobbly bit 'hanging loose' on your tummy. This includes loose skin which you can proudly call your 'twin skin' which may feel loose for months. You may also be a different shape to the shape you remember and feel your hips and pelvis may never get back into your favourite jeans. Gentle exercise is encouraged from the day after the birth and this definitely helps restore your shape. These exercises include slightly contracting your tummy muscles and building up strength gradually, in much the same way as you do your pelvic floor exercises.

Some mothers breastfeeding twins find their pregnancy weight just falls off while for others it won't budge. Breastfeeding hormones often work to protect fat stores in your body and dieting may not only be pointless, but harmful. Eat widely and wisely and enjoy it! If you're eating what you ate before you were pregnant, you'll be back to your pre-pregnancy weight within six months.

ANOTHER MUM SAYS   'I look at my jelly belly with pride and affection. I can wear those 'Bridget Jones' control briefs if I want to wear tight clothes.'

Abdominal separation

Abdominal separation can be experienced as pain or it can be a visible bulging of the separating muscles. It is caused by growth and hormones. It is advisable to exercise to put it back together. You may need to support your back using external support – seek professional advice from a women's health physio.

Exercises to do in hospital

- Pelvic floor muscle exercises – do these several times each day.
- Tighten your abdominal muscles for ten seconds while continuing to breathe normally.

- Rotate your feet and ankles, flexing and stretching your calves – this helps to avoid blood clots.
- Walk around the ward.
- Hold and cuddle your babies using techniques that are good for your back.
- Attend a postnatal physio class.

> ANOTHER MUM SAYS   'I didn't do my abdominal exercises and subsequently pulled a muscle in my tummy. The stomach muscles are really important as they primarily support your back.'

Post-partum blues

A few days after the birth, you will probably be feeling very, very emotional, happy, excited, weepy, upside down, moody, irritable, anxious, overjoyed, terrified ...

Most women experience a crash a few days after the euphoria of childbirth. The excitement and enormity of having their babies can make it difficult to sleep. Calling friends and having visitors, as well as looking after your babies, can suddenly get on top of you. Your hormone levels could also be going through some big changes. It is quite normal to find yourself crying uncontrollably all day or all week. Many women start crying the third day after the birth and cry all day or much longer. There may be many good reasons to cry, including:

- the early arrival of your babies
- your babies being admitted to the special care nursery
- your new role as parent
- the physical exhaustion of birth
- the pain during and following the birth
- struggling with the huge chasm between the birth you had imagined and the reality. It's quite common to grieve for the loss of that expectation.
- interrupted sleep or lack of sleep and having to wake to feed your babies
- the guilt of feeling ambivalent about your babies
- fear of not being able to look after them
- anxiety over your babies, their health, safety and their future
- the challenge of breastfeeding two babies
- the excitement of your babies arriving
- feeling overwhelmed by the responsibility and the emotions

Many women experience conflicting emotions at this time. It can be a time of great stress. Hospital is a safe place to feel miserable.

These feelings may pass quickly, may return sporadically or may not pass easily. If you're worried about the way you're feeling, talk to a professional. Take advantage of the services of the hospital. You may be feeling sad, anxious, depressed, disappointed, angry, scared, ambivalent ... anything. You may also feel joy, pleasure and love. Discussing the birth with anyone who'll listen will probably help you to absorb the reality of it. Your partner may remember things you didn't notice.

Post-partum psychosis symptoms are most likely to occur within 24–48 hours of your babies being born, so, while rare, it could happen in hospital. Medication is usually prescribed, with success.

See pages 204–213 for more information on depression.

(ANOTHER MUM SAYS)   'It was overwhelming having two of them to care for. I was sore and tired and feeling funny about breastfeeding. It was such a big effort, my nipples were squeezed by so many people and there was this building expectation, 'Has the milk come in yet?'

(ANOTHER MUM SAYS)   'The boys were pretty hungry and I was anxious that I wasn't giving them a good feed. One lovely midwife said, 'If I were you I'd give them a nice bottle and put them in the nursery so you all get a few hours sleep.' This really took the pressure off me and I also thought it was a great idea. The next day with them both feeding, my milk did come in a flood. It was a very emotional time and while I was extremely happy I was also crying over every meal. My husband was at first bemused and said, 'What's wrong, why aren't you happy?' and I blubbered through my chicken casserole that I'd never been so happy in my life. There they were, it was really happening. By the end of the week I was pushing my two babies around in their cribs proudly displaying my offspring and feeling ready to go home.'

Visitors

You may not know in advance whether you'll feel like having visitors, and it's fine to wait and see how it goes. Many mothers of twins find more people try to visit. Entertaining guests can be exhausting, even just talking can wear you out. While you may be keen to show your beautiful babies to the whole world, the world can also wait. Some strategies for controlling visitors in hospital:

- Let everyone know you'll be sticking to visiting hours only, or maybe having no visitors. Tell everyone to ring and check first.
- When visitors arrive, get your partner or the nurses to explain that while it's lovely to see them, you're all very tired and the *doctor* said visitors can only stay for *five minutes*.
- If visitors are outstaying their welcome *word up the staff* to come in and tell them you really need to rest *now*.
- Make signs to take to hospital with you: 'No visitors, please see nurses', 'Visitors in visiting hours only', 'Mother and babies sleeping, please do not disturb'.
- Decide not to have any visitors in hospital but organise an open day after you've been home for a week or so. Invite everyone to visit on that day, and suggest that they bring plenty to eat and drink.

If you have a 'no visitors' policy you might make one exception. New mums of twins can ask their hospital to contact AMBA or NZMBA (see page 340) as they can often arrange a hospital visitor. These hospital visitors are mothers of twins who volunteer to visit new twin mums and talk through any issues or concerns.

Helping your older children to cope
If you have older children, they will be going through an unsettling period where they are adjusting to lots of changes, many of which they won't like. While you're in hospital, there are things you can do to help them continue to feel an important part of the new family:

- Make sure someone else is holding the babies so your arms are free to hug and cuddle your children when they come to see you in hospital.
- Don't have the babies in your room at all when they visit.
- Introduce the babies as *their* new brothers and sisters rather than as *your* new babies.
- Let older children open any presents that arrive for the babies.
- Have some small gifts ready for your older children.

- Have activities like colouring books and puzzles handy.
- Speak to them on the phone while you're in hospital.
- Allow your children the opportunity to help you as much as possible.
- Show your children photos of them as babies, so they know they were once the subject of so much attention.
- Make sure they have a time to visit that is theirs alone, e.g. straight after school or kinder.

Bonding

Bonding is the emotional tug a parent feels for a young baby. Some parents fall in love with their babies during pregnancy or when they first see them, for others it never really happens for them. It isn't always easy to get to know one person at a time, so getting to know and love two can take longer. It can be confusing when, as soon as you lock your eyes on one baby, you are distracted by the other.

Many parents of twins report bonding with one baby instantly but not both, particularly if one baby is more challenging. If you don't fall in love with both your babies while you're in hospital, chances are that you will soon. Then again, some people say they didn't really love their children until they could walk and talk.

ANOTHER MUM SAYS 'Bonding with one of my boys took a little while, partly because I think I was a bit frightened of him. He was smaller than his brother and had been in Special Care so I didn't feel he was as robust. The first night he was with me he was lying down on the bed and was vomiting up through his nose and mouth. It was scary and left me a bit wary. No problem now, though. He's beautiful.'

Spending time with each baby separately can help. If your partner or midwives can attend to one baby for a while, you can spend time getting to know the other. There's no need to try too hard, it will probably just fall into place.

It has often been said that some twins are more identical than others, and the arrival of two babies at once can make it easy to get confused. It may take time but you'll work it out. You will probably notice differences in both their looks and personality fairly soon. Straight after their birth the hospital will 'tag' them on the wrist and perhaps the ankle too so everyone can tell who's who. Another way to tell them apart at a glance is to dress them differently. If your hospital is providing the clothes, you could ask for two different colours.

> (ANOTHER MUM SAYS)   'I remember reading that mothers learn very quickly to differentiate between when their baby is crying because she's hungry, in pain or is tired. Not only could I not tell the reason for crying, I also couldn't tell which baby was crying for the first three months. I had no time to think about differences, it all sounded the same to me, I just concentrated on what I needed to do next.'

If one or both of your babies are in Special Care or in an incubator, it may not be possible for you to cuddle and breastfeed them. This can make you feel anxious and sad, but there are still things you can do for your babies:

- Work towards establishing a supply of breastmilk.
- Spend time with the babies talking and singing to them.
- Touch or pat your babies through the portholes of the incubator.
- Take a video or photos of your babies.
- Ask staff what you can do to help care for them.

Low birth weight or pre-term babies sometimes don't look like the cute and cuddly babies you may have imagined. It is difficult to acknowledge not liking the look of your babies but don't panic, it's not uncommon. Newborn babies often have some features we may find unattractive, like fur and wrinkles, or they can look squashed. They will grow and change. Give them and yourself some time.

The death of a twin during pregnancy or soon after the birth often presents problems for the parents bonding with the survivor. Chapter 13 includes more discussion on this experience.

How long do I stay in hospital?

Many mothers of newborn twins find their hospital stay revolves around recovering from the birth and learning how to feed, bathe and change their babies. The midwives can be a great source of tips and information, but they may also have conflicting advice. Each one will do things a little differently, and this reinforces that there is no one right way to do things. In hospital it's easy to feel everyone but you knows what to do. It's the perfect time to listen and try out advice. In the end, you can decide what is best for you and yours.

It's easy to feel that you should just get on with it in hospital since you are going to have to cope alone at home, but hospital is the perfect place to rest and be waited on. Your health is important for looking after your babies. If you feel too tired, you can ask that your babies sleep in the nursery. If you want help, don't be afraid to press the buzzer.

All things being well, if you have a caesar you'll stay about a week; with a vaginal birth with twins you'll probably also stay a week. If you're sick of the hospital environment, try and spend a bit of time outdoors. A gentle walk in the fresh air or a 'pass out' (where the staff look after your babies while you leave the hospital) for a couple of hours may help.

Taking your babies home

Depending on how you feel and whether you think you're up to it, arrange for a family member or a close friend or neighbour to come around that afternoon or evening. Back in your home environment, you may be ready to see a familiar face and talk about your experience, as well as having a strong desire to show-off your beautiful new babies!

Alternatively, if you're not up to company, put your sign on the front door and turn the answering machine on. People can wait and they will understand that they will see you when you're ready. It's OK to focus on your new family right now.

Driving

Check with your medical insurer, who may insist you wait six weeks before driving following a caesarean. Even if you haven't had a caesarean, it's probably not a good idea to drive yourself home from hospital.

TIPS FOR SURVIVING YOUR HOSPITAL STAY

- Feel confident about asking for help – yours is a special situation.
- Have a notebook to write down your feeding times, questions and answers.
- Make a note of presents and their givers.
- If you don't understand what's happening, ask for explanations.
- Spend time with your babies.
- Spend some time with each baby one-on-one.
- Eat real food – get your favourites delivered, home-cooked or otherwise, if the hospital catering isn't up to scratch.
- You'll receive conflicting advice – make the most of the information you're being offered, but remember that you are the best person to decide what's right for you and your babies.
- Go to the hospital postnatal exercise class.
- Rest in hospital as much as you can, so that you'll have the energy to cope at home.

TIPS FOR PARTNERS

- Buy her chocolates, pick her flowers, make her a fresh fruit salad smoothie – or whatever she wants.
- Make the phone calls to let people know the news. Let them know your plans for visitors.
- Take lots of photos.
- Be at the hospital as much as you can to hold her hand and learn to change nappies and bathe babies.
- Organise grandparents or close friends to take older children overnight.
- Tell her what you're feeling.
- Ask her how she feels and listen to her reply (you don't have to fix it, just listening is great).
- Don't start talking about having another baby, yet!
- Cuddle your babies.
- If you can't be there, ring her a couple of times each day just to see how she's going.
- Have the house clean and tidy, food in the fridge and the evening meal ready for their arrival home.

The right support

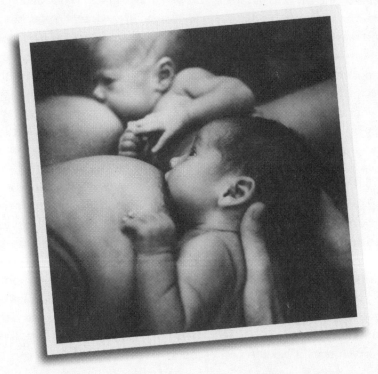

BREASTFEEDING

BREASTFEEDING: OUR STORIES

Breastfeeding your babies gives them the perfect food for their health and ongoing development. Most women, with help from their partners, and a range of health professionals, can successfully breastfeed their twins. Breastfeeding two babies works in the same way as breastfeeding one, and many mothers of twins continue to successfully breastfeed twins into their second year and beyond.

Katrina: I breastfed my twins for 14 months. I felt it was the healthiest option for my girls and myself. I knew breastmilk was the best food for my babies and they'd have fewer infections and allergies. I also thought it would give me freedom – if I was going out I could grab my babies and their nappy bag and head for the door.

When my babies were born the midwives encouraged my decision to breastfeed, and my babies latched on well from the start. I needed lots of help to manage each feed in the early stage. Breastfeeding was hard at the beginning, so much to master and remember while I was also recovering from major surgery. I needed help to attach them over and over again and the midwives were very patient. It was important that they helped me to do it, not do it for me. The main challenge for me was getting our positioning right so I could bring the babies to my breasts rather than trying to take my breasts to them. Each feed I alternated sides. To help remember which side was which I'd put a safety pin on my bra on the side Ella Hart had just been fed.

Once home I was able to feed both babies with my husband or my mother passing them to me. I took over the couch and propped the babies up to my breasts, with pillows under them and behind my back, to leave my hands free to use the remote control, read or eat while they fed. Hands-free meant I could also burp one baby mid-feed while the other kept feeding.

I made sure we were home at feed times for the first couple of months, unless I was at a trusted friend's home where they would prop us up with pillows in the bedroom and I could feed the babies together. I was determined to stick to the routine and keep their feeds synchronised. If one woke for a feed, I'd wake the other too.

The girls were six weeks old before I had to position them at the breast on my own. It was a juggling act to get propped up on the couch. Managing feeds on my own just got easier. Brad would get up each night to help me – he also found it a convenient hour to log on to the Internet.

After three months I was confident that feeding the babies separately once a day wouldn't upset their routine. It wasn't simple but at least I was out having coffee with the other mums! While I was feeding one I would push the pram back and forth with my foot to keep the other happy.

At first the girls were feeding for about an hour out of every three, but after six months it only took them 10 minutes. They were becoming stronger suckers and were getting bigger so were able to fit more in their tummies.

At one stage I had so much milk rushing out that the girls would cough and splutter. For a few days I expressed milk for five minutes before each feed. This relieved the pressure of my milk let down and the girls could attach happily. It also meant I built up a stash of breastmilk in the freezer for the girls if I wanted to go out without them.

I had a huge appetite and ate constantly. My weight fell off and I was soon slimmer than my pre-pregnancy weight. I thought it would be good if I could breastfeed them forever. As the girls started eating real food they gradually dropped breastfeeds themselves. At 14 months it was down to one feed at bedtime. I was ready to give it up but at the same time reluctant to let that last feed go. I wanted them to 'need' their mummy and I liked the feeling that my milk was the best thing for them. But I became quite sick and didn't have the energy to feed them. Their dad gave them a bottle of cow's milk at bedtime.

I'm very proud of myself for breastfeeding for 14 months, and realise I succeeded mostly because my partner and family supported me.

Louise: When I was six months pregnant I went to see a breastfeeding consultant to get some tips on breastfeeding two babies at once. She gave me lots to read and a lesson on how to express colostrum. I knew from ultrasound scans that one of my babies was a lot smaller than the other and was likely to be admitted to Special Care when born. So I decided to express colostrum drop by drop while I was pregnant and freeze it for my small baby to be given when he or she arrived. I collected it in those wee sample jars and had two half-full, which I had put in to the nursery freezer when I arrived at the hospital.

Celeste did need to go in to Special Care when she was born to have her temperature monitored. She was fed my expressed colostrum through a tube in her nose. Midwives were in and out of my room constantly, wanting to know how I'd thought to express colostrum and telling me what a great idea it was.

Camille went straight to my breast when I came out of recovery. She latched on easily. After the first night the girls were ready for me to feed them together. I sat up in bed with heaps of pillows to balance us all. There were visitors and a couple of midwives there to help us. Once on, it was more comfortable than I had imagined. I found it embarrassing though, to be so exposed. Both breasts at once felt like I was topless in the middle of winter while everyone around me was fully clothed and fascinated. If I had my time again, I'd insist on no visitors in those first few days.

After a couple of days, rather than feeding on the bed, I sat in a big lounge chair in my hospital room surrounded by pillows. I needed help from a midwife to bring the girls to me one by one and latch them on. Then the midwife would leave the room. A couple of times I got stranded either forgetting to have the buzzer nearby or buzzing and getting no reply. I was very sensitive at this stage, a post-operative first time mother of twins, upset and stuck holding two crying babies with no one to help.

When I got home I sat in a big low leather chair with armrests. We didn't have a couch. I collected the girls one by one putting each on a bouncer next to my chair. This made them high enough for me to pick them up one at a time quite easily.

Celeste, being a lot smaller, was slower. Once I had mastered it, I could never get the hang of anything but the 'underarm hold'. Even feeding them one at a time felt awkward, I felt like they were facing the wrong way.

The girls continued to have some formula from a bottle after each breastfeed. It was so much more time-consuming doing both breast and bottle every feed than if they'd just been breastfed. They weren't getting enough with just breastmilk so I battled on. In retrospect, I should've seen the breastfeeding consultant after the girls were born and tried to increase my supply. Having spoken to many other twin mothers who also breastfed, expressed and bottle-fed, I think getting professional advice early can interrupt that vicious cycle of continuing to add formula and, as a result, decreasing milk supply.

After nine weeks I wasn't getting any sleep. The most sleep I'd had in a row in months was two and a half hours. If I bottle-fed I could feed them both in just under an hour. This idea had a lot of appeal. I remember calculating in my head how many weeks of breastmilk they'd had and whether I could justify stopping yet.

I stopped breastfeeding when I took the girls to 'sleep school' at nine weeks. The nurses bottle fed them overnight and I slept and slept.

How does breastfeeding work?

During pregnancy your breasts may become larger or firmer as the glands prepare to produce milk for your babies. Your nipples may look darker and feel tender. You might notice colostrum, a thick, yellowish fluid coming from your nipples. Colostrum is rich in antibodies and protects your babies from disease. Your milk production usually increases dramatically (the milk 'comes in') within a week of the birth of your babies and becomes a thin, bluish-white milk. Your babies suckle at the breast, stimulating the nerves in your nipples. Hormones are then released into your bloodstream, activating the milk making tissues and causing the breast to push out or 'let down' the milk. At each feed your babies begin by sucking rapidly, then when the milk lets down they move to a slower, more rhythmic swallow. When your babies drink milk, your breasts make more milk to replace it. If the milk isn't removed the milk production will slow down.

Breastfeeding twins

Given the right support and advice almost all mothers of twins can breastfeed their babies. It is widely recognised that babies should be exclusively breastfed for six months. Some of the reasons you may want to breastfeed your babies are:

- Breastmilk is the perfect food for your babies. The composition of your breastmilk constantly changes to the right ingredients according to what your babies need.
- Breastmilk is safe for your babies and is easy for them to digest.
- Breastmilk is always available when your babies need it.
- Breastmilk doesn't cost anything and doesn't take any time to prepare.
- Breastfeeding two babies means that no one else can feed them so you can rest while feeding.
- Breastfeeding helps you to adjust to motherhood and feel close to your babies with plenty of time for looking, cuddling and close contact.
- Your babies absorb the nutrients, so they can grow and develop to their full potential.

- Your babies' immune systems are strengthened by breast milk so they have less sickness and fewer allergies, which also means less expense on doctors' bills and medication.
- Breastfeeding assists your babies' brain development as breastmilk contains essential amino acids not found in formula.
- Breastfeeding may help you lose weight more quickly after the birth.

Preparing to breastfeed your twins

No special nipple preparation is needed before your babies are born but there are some things you may like to do to prepare yourself to breast-feed your twins:

- Go, preferably with your partner, to a breastfeeding for beginners class.
- Go, preferably with your partner, to a breastfeeding consultant for information and advice.
- Buy a couple of maternity bras, making sure they're comfortable and easy to undo. Getting fitted by an expert means you won't make an expensive mistake. They are more likely to know how much your breasts will grow, so will fit you with your correct size and shape.
- Learn some breathing and relaxation exercises, relaxing helps your milk to be made available more easily.
- Eat good nutritious food.
- Visit and talk with a counsellor at Australian Breastfeeding Association (Australia) or La Leche League (New Zealand). They give advice and sell booklets on breastfeeding twins.
- Get in touch with your local multiple birth club and meet other mothers who have successfully breastfed twins.
- Discuss your desire to breastfeed and what you are learning with your partner and ask for support and encouragement.
- Find someone who has successfully breastfed twins and who is happy to stay in contact and support and encourage you through the difficult times.

Learning to breastfeed

In hospital you will probably be encouraged to feed your babies as soon as possible after their birth. Babies' suckling reflexes are strongest straight after birth so if you put your babies to the breast as soon as possible they will begin to stimulate your breasts to produce milk. For your first breastfeeds the midwives will help you to position and attach your babies at the breast. They will give you advice about different positions for simultaneous feeding or separate feeding, and will support you in working out what suits you best. Many mothers use a number of ways to breastfeed their babies. You could use a few different ways at different ages and stages of breastfeeding.

ANOTHER MUM SAYS   'It was so difficult, the babies were screaming with hunger and I was about to start them on formula. My twin sister was breastfeeding her six-month-old and offered to give my babies a lesson. It proved to me that the babies have to learn to breastfeed too. It was amazing, one feed from her and they both latched on to me for their next feed and never looked back.'

Breastfeeding babies other than your own is acceptable – sometimes it can be of great benefit in an emergency – providing that you are not taking any medications or recreational drugs, and that you and the baby you are feeding are in good health and are free of infection.

ANOTHER MUM SAYS   'One of my girls continued to struggle with breastfeeding for about the first month and has never had the same weight gains as the other. But she is a perfectly happy baby, and even on solids has never put on huge amounts of weight.'

ANOTHER MUM SAYS   'The first six to eight weeks were a bit of a blur. My fantastic husband took the first seven weeks off, so was at home to help carry babies to and from their bassinettes and to help settle them, as well as to do the washing and housework. After that it got easier. It gets easier after the first eight weeks whether you breastfeed or not.'

'When things aren't going well, weaning is often the only solution people offer. People may tell you that breastfeeding twins takes a lot out of you, but so does standing at the sink for an hour a day preparing bottles.'
AMBA lactation consultant

The difference when breastfeeding two babies rather than one is the positioning of your babies if you're feeding them simultaneously (both at the breast at the same time) and the amount of time spent breastfeeding if you're feeding them separately.

Positioning and attachment

At antenatal classes and in hospital, your midwife will teach you how to position and attach your babies. It also helps to watch other people, visit a breastfeeding consultant and to speak to someone from the ABA or La Leche League (New Zealand).

How long does it take to breastfeed two babies?

It is normal for a breastfed baby to feed between six and 12 times in 24 hours. It usually takes between 10 and 30 minutes for a baby to feed, but this is just a rough guide. It can take longer. Your two babies may have completely different appetites and preferences, which is fine.

> ANOTHER MUM SAYS   'My small babies took at least 45 minutes for each feed (and sometimes up to an hour and a quarter) for about the first three to four months. But by treating this time as a rest and a special cuddle time, it did not worry me. I had a table next to me with lots of essential things on it – a water bottle, a bowl of fruit, books, magazines and the television remote control, so this time was like a break from an otherwise often hectic day. It also meant that visitors who came and offered to help could do things like bring in washing and fold it or help with dinner. I'm sure if I had been bottle-feeding I would have had plenty of volunteers to feed the babies and I would have been left with the other jobs.'

How much do they need?

If you are concerned that your babies are not getting enough breastmilk, check that:

- Your babies have six to eight pale wet cloth nappies in 24 hours, or five heavily wet disposable nappies.
- Your babies are alert and generally happy, and have good skin colour.
- They are growing in weight, length and head circumference. It is quite normal for your twins to be different and to grow at different rates and times.

You may mistakenly think your milk supply is low if:

- Your breasts feel less full. Your supply may have settled down once your milk started flowing well, although you feel less full than you did when you first started to breastfeed.
- Your babies want more frequent feeds. This may be due to your babies' increased appetite, rather than your milk supply dropping. Feeding more often will build up your supply to meet their need.
- Your babies begin to feed really quickly.
- Your babies are unwell or unsettled and are feeding more frequently. If your babies have stuffy noses or sore throats they may prefer to have lots of small feeds, just to cover their hunger, but not a full feed, as feeding may not be comfortable.
- They want lots of quick feeds in hot weather to quench their thirst rather than to fill up.
- Your babies' weight gains slow down. Babies weight gains can fluctuate.

If you think your babies are not getting enough breastmilk, seek expert advice on how to increase your milk production.

> (ANOTHER MUM SAYS) 'Weight gain was probably the biggest issue with my babies. Like many breastfed babies, their gains were erratic, and they have never really had a period of huge gains. This concerned their paediatrician for a while, but even he was eventually satisfied that they were very healthy, happy and contented babies who met all their developmental milestones. After one visit to the health centre when neither had put on much weight I went to an Australian Breastfeeding Association meeting and they were just great. They reassured me that weight gains can be erratic but as long as everything else is OK, the babies are fine and are getting all the benefits of breastfeeding. I recently read a book about child nutrition that stated that at one year of age breastfed babies as a group are smaller than their bottle-fed counterparts. It also said that as growth charts are based on American data from the 1960s and 1970s when most babies were bottle-fed they are not necessarily the best guide for breastfed babies.'

Standard growth charts are based on weights and heights of single babies. Twins can take up to six years to catch up.

SOME IDEAS TO MAKE MORE BREASTMILK

- Make sure you're getting enough rest and good nutritious food.
- If you're in pain after the birth, talk to your doctor about managing your pain.
- Check the babies are positioned correctly at the breast.
- Allow the babies to stay on the breast for as long as they want.
- Offer the breast instead of a dummy for a while to increase your milk production.
- Express half an hour or so after a feed. The added stimulation helps increase milk. It may take a couple of days to notice the increase.
- If feeding your babies separately, then try feeding them together. The milk let down can be stronger when two babies are suckling together.
- Talk to a breastfeeding expert or counsellor at La Leche League (New Zealand) or the Australian Breastfeeding Association.

Appetite increases

It can happen at any time, but at six weeks, three months and six months babies often have a sudden increase in appetite. With twins it can happen to both babies simultaneously or at different times. One or both babies may suddenly be unsettled, wake earlier, and want to feed more often than usual for a few days then may settle back into their old pattern. Letting them feed as often as they want to will increase your supply to meet their need. Many women worry that their supply has dropped but find when they listen to their babies and feed more frequently their milk supply adjusts within the week.

'Many women start off breastfeeding but hit the wall when the babies are about six weeks old. They're often physically exhausted, locked onto the couch all day feeding, while their partner is standing around feeling like a spare wheel. They're twisted in knots and the emotional attachment often makes it such a difficult decision.'
AMBA home visitor

ANOTHER MUM SAYS 'When my babies' appetites increase I take them to bed with me. I rest and feed them whenever I can.'

'Many women with single babies also reach crisis point at six weeks. The problem often occurs then because the babies go through an appetite increase at six weeks and need more milk. That's when the mother needs to offer more feeds to build up her milk supply. It can take a few days for the system to kick in but usually then things will improve. Women often start to take the mini-pill around the six-week mark which can also affect milk supply.'
AMBA breastfeeding consultant

ANOTHER MUM SAYS 'At three and a half months, I nearly stopped breastfeeding. I was physically exhausted and they seemed to want to feed more often. I went to a Breastfeeding Association meeting on breastfeeding twins and was inspired by a woman half my size who had only just finished feeding her 15-month-old boys. She inspired me to continue. From what I can gather many mums stop at this time. My advice is to seek out other breastfeeding mums to get your second wind.'

Twin feeding

Many mothers of twins are unsure about whether to begin twin feeding from the very first breastfeed, especially if these are their first babies. Feeding both of your babies at the same time can seem a little awkward at first but can be very relaxing once you've all mastered the technique.

If you are feeding simultaneously there will probably be times where one baby wakes and is hungry, so you need to wake the other in order to feed them together. Most babies adapt fairly quickly to being woken to feed together.

Feeding separately

In an ideal world each baby is fed on their own schedule, feeding when they're hungry. Some mothers don't want to wake their second baby to feed or may find their baby doesn't feed well after being woken. Some mothers don't like the idea of waking a sleeping baby or you may have one baby that needs to be fed more frequently than the other.

ANOTHER MUM SAYS 'I fed to need overnight for two weeks and nearly went mad. I thought it might encourage my babies to sleep for longer. I'd feed one then as soon as my head hit the pillow the other baby would wake to be fed. I went back to twin feeding so I could sleep when they did.'

ANOTHER MUM SAYS   'I tried to feed the babies together because I liked the idea of saving time but I never really enjoyed it. I have continued to this day to feed them individually when they want it. On a few occasions I have woken one baby up overnight so I could feed them one after the other just to get a little more sleep. It has been a bit hairy on occasions when they've both needed feeding at once but I used a rocker at my feet to amuse one while the other fed.'

Breastfeeding your twins separately but one straight after the other means both babies are in the same routine. You may find separate feeding easier until the babies have head control. If both babies want to feed at the same time, it can be difficult to relax and feed one baby while the other is crying. It can also be difficult to settle the baby you've just fed while the second baby is crying. A pram, bouncinette or baby swing can be very useful at these times.

ANOTHER MUM SAYS   'Feeding my twins has been two different experiences. One has always been very matter of fact, breastfed quickly and then settled into his cot and slept alone, whereas the other has fed and fed and fed.'

ANOTHER MUM SAYS   'I had a five-and-a-half-year-old and a three-year-old when my twins were born and I found it was often easier to feed them separately. In the mornings I'd have one in a bouncer on the kitchen floor and one feeding, then swap over. It meant I could feed while I answered the phone, buttered toast, tied a shoelace, wiped a nose. It also helped that my twins were quite quick feeders from the start, taking around 25 minutes. I didn't expect they would necessarily feed the same, as my two others had been very different feeders.'

Combining simultaneous feeding and separate feeding

You can experiment with simultaneous feeding and feeding separately to see what suits you and your babies. You may prefer to feed simultaneously during the day, then feed separately at night, encouraging your babies to sleep longer overnight. Or to feed separately during the day, then get more sleep yourself overnight by feeding simultaneously.

If one or both of your babies are unsettled or unwell, you may prefer to feed them separately for a while so you can concentrate while it's difficult.

ANOTHER MUM SAYS   'For the first six or seven months I mostly fed my babies together – waking the other when one woke for a feed. But their last evening feed was usually separate, and this final separate feed is still part of their bedtime routine. As they reduced the number of feeds they needed each day and as they fed faster, I fed them separately more often.'

One breast each or alternating each feed?

You will work out what suits you and your babies. Some mothers find one baby doesn't suck as strongly so they alternate breasts at each feed to build up their milk supply in both breasts. Some women's breasts have different milk producing abilities so they prefer to swap sides regularly. It also helps the babies get different visual stimulation if they feed on different sides. Others find that when their babies have different feeding needs, they prefer to feed them on the same side so each breast adapts to the needs of one baby.

Simultaneous feeding positions

Many women use different positions for breastfeeding in different locations. Try the bed, the couch, the floor, a comfy chair, a futon against a wall, a bean bag . . . whatever works best for you. In bed you might feed your babies while you're reclining. Plenty of cushions and pillows are always handy. It is important that you're all comfortable, but keep in mind it's unsafe for babies to fall asleep on adult pillows.

Underarm hold: The underarm hold is the most popular simultaneous feeding position. It is the easiest position to get into if you don't have help, it works well for small babies and it leaves your hands free. If you've had a caesarean it puts less pressure on your wound.

- Have 6 pillows handy. Lie one pillow each side of where you sit.
- Lie the babies where you can reach them safely while sitting.
- Sit with your feet on a footstool or with pillows under your knees.
- Lie your babies with their heads on pillows in your lap, with their legs extended under your arms and their faces facing yours.
- One at a time, cup each baby's head in your hands and lift it to your breast. Hug the babies close to you with your elbow.
- Raise your knees to a height where the babies heads are supported at the right height without you crouching over.

The parallel hold: The parallel hold works better with older babies, and is convenient when feeding away from home as you don't need piles of pillows. It can also be more discreet but can be difficult if they kick each other.

- Hold the first baby as you would if breastfeeding one baby.
- Lean the second baby on, and parallel to, the first. One baby's body supports the head of the other while you hold them both in position.
- Raise your knees to a height that means you don't have to crouch over.

Crisscross hold: The crisscross hold is difficult with weaker feeders and smaller babies. It can also be more difficult until they have some head control at around six weeks.

- Place the heavier baby in the single breastfeeding position.
- Gently lie the second baby across the first so they are crisscrossed facing each other.
- Support their backs with your arms and clasp your hands under their bottoms to bring them closer to you.

V-hold: The V-hold can be a useful position for feeding your babies at night as you can stay in a semi lying down position and doze. It can also be helpful after a vaginal delivery if sitting is uncomfortable. Again it's difficult when babies are under about six weeks old as they don't have much head control. Support your back with pillows.

- Put a baby to each breast so they are facing each other and their knees are bent and touching.
- Support their backs with your arms while your hands cup their bottoms.

Breastfeeding away from home

If you always feed your babies simultaneously, you might continue to do this if you are visiting friends or family and can set yourself up comfortably. When you're out in public, simultaneous feeding can be awkward, so many mothers feed their twins separately when out. If you feed them separately, you may need to keep your other baby entertained with a toy, a dummy, cuddles from a friend or by rocking the pram with your foot.

Burping your babies

Burping helps your babies bring up any air they have swallowed while drinking. The wind can cause tummy pains in some babies, while other babies don't need burping at all. It can be a bit awkward burping two babies at once but if you do need to burp both babies, you could try:

- lying them on their tummies with a pillow under their chests, then propping them up one at a time and gently rubbing their backs
- sitting them up one at a time while the other continues to feed
- lie one on their tummy while you prop the other on your shoulder

Night feeding

Night feeds help to build and maintain your milk supply. Accepting that your babies will probably wake, rather than resenting it when they do, can make night feeding less stressful.

- Try to let your babies know it is night-time, keeping the house quiet and dark. This helps with settling back to sleep with as little fuss as possible.
- Simultaneous feeding is quicker but may mean you are waking a baby who would otherwise sleep longer.
- Feeding one after the other (waking the second baby) means you may then have a nice stretch of sleep.
- You could try feeding to need and dozing or falling asleep while feeding each baby, settling the first back in her cot when the second one wakes, then dozing off as you feed her.
- Using disposable nappies overnight means you may not need to change them.
- Your partner may be able to bring the babies to you and settle them back in their cots when they finish feeding. This makes night feeding easier.

ANOTHER MUM SAYS   'One night I stopped waking the second baby for the feed and she slept through.'

Expressing

This is explained in detail on pages 275–278.

Potential problems

Nipple care

You may experience nipple tenderness when you first begin to breastfeed. Your nipples may be more sensitive for the first few days after the birth of your babies. You are learning how to breastfeed and so are your babies. Attaching your babies correctly, positioning them properly, and taking care when you take them off the breast, all take time and patience to learn. If feeding is painful, your babies may not be attached properly. To avoid this pain and to prevent further problems, get professional help from your midwife, maternal child health centre, ABA or La Leche (New Zealand).

AVOIDING AND HEALING SORE NIPPLES

- Make sure the babies are correctly positioned and attached.
- There is no need to wash your nipples before or after feeding.
- There is no need to put any creams or ointment on your nipples.
- Don't try to harden or toughen your nipples with brushes or methylated spirits.
- Washing your nipples with soap is unnecessary and may dry them out.
- After feeds, hand-express a few drops of milk and smear on your nipples and allow to dry.
- If you need to re-attach your babies, break the suction first by inserting your clean finger in your babies' mouths.
- Air-dry your nipples. Don't tuck them back into your bra while they're still wet. Change nursing pads often to keep your nipples dry and prevent infection.

Seek expert advice if you are considering expressing for a while to give your nipples a rest. If your nipples become sore, very red, bruised or blistered, seek expert advice.

Cracked or sore nipples can also be caused by:
- incorrect attachment – your babies are sucking on the nipple rather than the areola. If the baby's grip on your breast feels painful, pop a clean finger in the corner of his or her mouth, break the suction, then try again.
- thrush – a fungal infection that usually needs an antithrush treatment to clear it up
- dermatitis – seek medical advice

Cracked nipples usually make feeding painful and may start to bleed. Correct positioning and attachment will help the nipple heal. Treatment is the same as for sore nipples. If it's too painful, seek expert advice on how to express your milk by hand until the crack starts to heal.

Blocked ducts

If you have any sore spot on your breasts, the sooner you start treatment the better. If left, it can develop into an infection. A blocked milk duct can make part of your breast red, lumpy or swollen, feeling tender and painful. This can happen at any stage of breastfeeding. Try the following for relief:

- Changing the position of your baby for a feed can help to clear a blocked duct.
- Try feeding more frequently from that breast to empty as much milk as possible.
- Apply heat with a hot flannel before feeding.
- Gently massage the affected area toward the nipple during and after feeds.
- If your breast is still sore after 12 hours see your doctor or breastfeeding consultant.
- See if you can work out the cause – it could be pressure from clothing, an ill-fitting bra or a hand supporting the breast while you are feeding. Keeping your bra off at night and slipping the bra cup off completely while feeding can help as this will stop the bra putting pressure on a duct.

Mastitis

This breast inflammation or infection can occur when a milk duct in the breast becomes blocked, or following a cracked nipple. It can make you feel unwell, with a high temperature, hot and cold fevers or you may have a red tender patch on your breast. It can be very painful.

- See your doctor as soon as possible. You will probably need an antibiotic.
- Keep feeding from the breast as this will also help you to get better.
- Make sure your maternity bras fit properly.
- It's an infection so it's also important to rest to help your body heal itself.

(ANOTHER MUM SAYS) 'I breastfed my first child so I put pressure on myself to breastfeed the twins. I nearly gave up after two bouts of mastitis, but I'm glad I didn't because it became so easy and convenient.'

Thrush

When you are breastfeeding and taking antibiotics, the chances of you and the babies developing thrush increase. Thrush is a fungus and it thrives on milk in warm moist situations. It can also develop following a cracked nipple and can be a nuisance as well as causing pain. It may appear as persistent nappy rash on the babies or as white spots inside their mouths. Your doctor will probably suggest a treatment for you and your babies. Remember to use it according to instructions, otherwise the thrush can recur.

(ANOTHER MUM SAYS) 'When I started taking antibiotics for mastitis, my paediatrician recommended putting an oral thrush medicine on my nipples before feeding the babies. It worked.'

Keeping your energy levels up

Eat, eat, eat. This is the recommended daily intake when you breastfeed twins but you may need to eat more according to your appetite.

DAIRY: 5 serves
    1 serve = 1 cup milk
    1 serve = 1 cup cottage cheese
    1 serve = 1 slice hard cheese

MEAT, FISH, POULTRY AND EGGS: 2 serves

FRESH VEGETABLES: 4 cups (2 cups cooked)

FRUIT: 2–3 pieces

BREAD AND CEREALS: at least 4–5 serves

BUTTER OR OIL: 2 tablespoons

You need to eat lots when you're breastfeeding twins and you may even be hungry after eating a meal. Hopefully groceries will be home-delivered so there is always fresh food in the house. There may not always be a casserole on the doorstep, so you need quick, easy one-handed food.

- Try to keep plenty of food in the house that you can grab quickly from the fridge or freezer with one hand and heat up in the microwave (soups, pasties, meal-size portions of curry and rice or casserole).
- Sleep and rest. Sit down and put your feet up when you can.
- Exercise gives you energy. It needn't be vigorous. Try putting your babies in the pram and taking them for a walk.

NUTRITIOUS ONE-HANDED SNACK FOODS
cheese and vegemite sandwiches
fresh fruit, cut up ready to grab from the fridge
dried fruit
cheese and biscuits
yoghurt
milk shakes and smoothies
boiled eggs
raw vegetables
cups of soup
pieces of quiche
baked beans and tinned spaghetti
biscuits with cream cheese
Turkish bread and dips

Foods to avoid when breastfeeding
Most mothers can eat any foods in moderation. You may like to avoid foods that you know you or your partner are allergic to and it may be prudent to avoid foods that you dislike or that disagree with you. You might find that your babies get upset if you eat excessive amounts of some foods. Elimination followed by the introduction of suspected offending foods may be tried. Dairy foods, chocolate, oranges, wheat and onions are among the foods sometimes considered to cause problems. Drinks containing caffeine can also upset your baby particularly if consumed in large quantities.

Support from your partner

Support from your partner can have an enormous influence on your ability to manage breastfeeding. An encouraging partner is usually tired, stressed and confused too, yet many partners are happy to get up and collect babies for feeds overnight and then settle them back to bed after the feed. This type of help is invaluable.

> (ANOTHER MUM SAYS) 'I am still feeding my 13-month-old girls twice a day. Breastfeeding twins can bring a special joy. My mornings start with my husband bringing the two girls to our bed for their morning feed. It's lovely to have the pair of them tucked into my sides for a relaxed feed to start the day.'

> (ANOTHER MUM SAYS) 'My partner has been unbelievable. Every time the babies woke overnight for a feed he got them from the cots and brought them to me in bed and then returned them to the cots when they were finished. I feel truly blessed and would never have been able to breastfeed so successfully without him.'

Breastfeeding twins when you have a toddler

Breastfeeding your twins when you have a toddler gives you an opportunity to sit down and rest when perhaps you otherwise wouldn't.

If you are feeding simultaneously, you won't be able to move, so here are some ideas you may like to try to help things run as smoothly as possible:

- Make sure your house is childproof or that you can close off the room to keep your toddler with you.
- Check he or she can get to the toilet if they need to, or take them before you get yourself set up.
- Have within your reach snacks, toys, books, videos and the remote control, plus anything else you or your child might need.
- Feed in a position that allows you to have a hand or two free to touch or play with your toddler.
- Feeding your toddler his meal at the same time may work, so have everything set up and ready.

- Put a mattress or couch in the room where you feed so you can also lie down and maybe doze off while older children are playing.
- Organise a breastfeed to coincide with your toddler napping beside you or resting beside you with a book.
- Try to plan an activity to do with your toddler between feeds: playdough, painting or baking a cake.
- Try to organise a baby-sitter between feeds occasionally so you can take your toddler swimming, shopping, dancing, even if it's just for an hour.
- Talk with other mothers breastfeeding twins who have a toddler, and share your experiences and ideas.

ANOTHER MUM SAYS   'One of my greatest concerns about having a young and active child and newborn twins was breastfeeding. Determined to feed the babies myself, I did obtain a book about breastfeeding twins and read it while I was pregnant. Ideally, I would be feeding them together and we bought a sofa for their room for that purpose. I would be confined to their bedroom with my three-year-old on a four hourly basis. While this is a concern for all mothers with toddlers who are breastfeeding, breastfeeding twins is far more restrictive. You must have pillows for support, and be on a large chair or couch. With one baby it's quite easy to follow your toddler/child around the house, or outside for that matter. I found this the most frustrating aspect of breastfeeding twins.'

ANOTHER MUM SAYS   'The activity box was supposed to be the solution to my problem. The idea is to fill a box with all kinds of new and interesting toys/activities for the older sibling. Ideally, they become so preoccupied with this box that mother and babies sit back blissfully to feed and bond. My activity box lasted a week. I really needed other distractions such as videos and storybooks. I eventually became clever enough to read to my daughter while breastfeeding. As the twins got bigger, I didn't need my hands to hold them in place as much and I was freed-up to turn pages, brush hair and shake my finger disapprovingly at naughty antics.'

Becoming pregnant with twins while breastfeeding

It's a good idea to talk to your toddler about sharing breastfeeding with the new baby. If you become pregnant with twins while breastfeeding an older child, your milk supply may decrease. You may decide to wean at this time or you may choose to continue to feed. Ask your medical adviser to check your iron levels as being pregnant while breastfeeding can contribute to low iron levels. If you are hospitalised, it can be comforting for your toddler to have breastfeeds while visiting you in hospital.

Often the newborn feeds differently and more frequently than the toddler. Breastfeeding your toddler may not reduce the tenderness sometimes felt during the early days of breastfeeding a newborn, however a toddler can help to relieve any engorgement.

(ANOTHER MUM SAYS) 'My most memorable breastfeeding experience would have to be when I brought the babies home for the first time. My daughter asked if she could have a go so I fed her (a three-year-old) and a newborn together. Those two faces looking up at me were just heaven on a stick. That was the last feed our daughter ever had.'

(ANOTHER MUM SAYS) 'My two-and-a-half-year-old daughter was still breastfeeding twice a day when I conceived twins. At 23 weeks I was hospitalised for the remainder of my pregnancy but continued to breastfeed her when she visited most days. My supply dropped and changed to colostrum and I wondered when she might lose interest, but she continued to feed, even the night before her sisters were born at 36 weeks by caesarean. She was delighted watching the babies breastfeed and she waited until we all came home before meekly asking if she could have a turn after the babies had fed. Feeding the twins is a wonderful experience and at six months they are still exclusively breastfed, with my daughter having a little turn most days.'

Weaning

Weaning is the process of introducing foods other than breastmilk into your babies' diet. You may reach a point where you want to decrease the number of breastfeeds per day, or you may want to stop altogether. Often well-meaning friends and family suggest you wean before you're ready, suggesting breastfeeding two babies is too draining or time-consuming. You may also feel pressure to continue to breastfeed. You and your babies are the best ones to decide when weaning is right for you.

ANOTHER MUM SAYS 'It's been hard dealing with comments from family members such as 'You're not still feeding those babies are you?' While people are quick to make such comments, I find it frustrating that they don't seem to make the connection that breastfeeding has meant very few illnesses and the babies have met all their developmental milestones. I have no plans to stop breastfeeding my babies. I'll let them do it in their own time. In the meantime I couldn't think of anything I'd rather be doing than sitting down relaxing and breastfeeding a baby.'

When you begin to wean your babies, they will take less breastmilk and your body will adjust and make less milk. Gradual weaning is best for you and your babies, so it's ideal if you don't have the pressure of a time limit. Gradual weaning means you have less likelihood of engorged breasts, your hormone changes are less severe and your babies are able to continue feeling secure.

Weaning twins is almost the same as weaning one baby.

- You may find that cutting out a breastfeed is sometimes the best way to continue breastfeeding your babies, rather than stopping completely.
- Sometimes one twin may choose to wean earlier than the other. This is fine. Don't feel that because you are weaning one baby you must wean them both.
- Watch out for blocked ducts and mastitis even if one of your babies is still feeding. Check regularly for lumps and express milk if necessary to avoid blocked ducts or a breast infection.

ANOTHER MUM SAYS 'I was starting to feel quite exhausted when our babies were three months old. We decided my partner would give the babies a bottle of formula at their 11 p.m. feed. I started going to bed at 9 p.m. and sleeping till 3 a.m. Because I consistently had six hours then another two hours sleep every night, I managed to continue breastfeeding for another three months. I'm glad we came up with this solution and I could continue to breastfeed rather than wean.'

Planned weaning is when you make the decision to wean. It involves introducing your babies to a bottle or a cup. Start by not offering the babies the breastfeed they seem least interested in throughout the day, then cut out each feed gradually.

What you replace your babies' breastfeeds with will depend on the age of your babies. Discuss this with your medical adviser. The general rule is:
- formula for babies younger than 12 months
- cows milk for babies 12 months or older

If one or both of your babies seems reluctant to wean try:
- Offering the bottle at the feed at which they're likely to be hungriest.
- Giving formula before offering a breastfeed.
- Feeding to a routine.
- Giving your babies a dummy for comfort sucking.
- Changing your routine, perhaps going out and offering a cup or bottle rather than a breastfeed.
- Leaving the room, or the house, for half an hour while someone else offers the bottle.
- Asking your partner to resettle the babies at night.
- Asking your partner to feed the babies formula.

ANOTHER MUM SAYS   'At first I thought it was a problem that my son didn't want to give up the breast, but it wasn't. It was just what he needed as an individual. His twin brother was always ambivalent about the boobs. So you have to take each baby as they come and work out what's best for all of you. Don't let anyone tell you that you're letting your children down by doing it this way or that way. They're not the ones that have to deal with it. I was a little sad to give breastfeeding away, that time was over, and a bit guilty (but it didn't last long) but I knew it was the best thing for all of us. I was proud I'd got that far.'

Your emotions when weaning

Many mothers continue to breastfeed until their babies wean themselves. Your emotions can be complex if your babies are ready to wean but you would like to continue breastfeeding.

Even if you are very keen to wean, your feelings may surprise you. Many women feel sad, weepy and even depressed after their last feed. Your hormones need to adjust to their pre-pregnancy and pre-lactating levels and this can take some time. You may also be grieving for that very close and constant relationship with your babies. Talking to other mothers who have breastfed or a counsellor from the Australian Breastfeeding Association or La Leche League (New Zealand) will reassure you.

TIPS FOR SUCCESSFUL BREASTFEEDING

- Visit a breastfeeding consultant or go to a breastfeeding class while you are pregnant.
- Subscribe to the Australian Breastfeeding Association. Their information and support can be invaluable when you start breastfeeding.
- Watch and observe other mothers breastfeeding twins, preferably while you're pregnant.
- Make sure your babies are properly attached to the breast and that you're comfortable.
- Drink plenty of water and eat plenty of nutritious food.
- Keep food, drinks, the phone and the remote control near you when feeding.
- Accept genuinely helpful offers to clean, cook and childmind. Avoid people who cause tension or create work.
- Rest and relax at every opportunity, particularly when your babies are sleeping.
- Breathe deeply and remember that you're doing a fantastic job.
- Have a regular massage.
- Take one day at a time ... this time next year they'll be walking to the kitchen for their dinner.

TIPS FOR PARTNERS

- Make it easier for her by changing the babies before their feed.
- Even though you can't actually feed the babies, be involved in breastfeeding – burp the babies during and after feeds.
- Take things to her while she breastfeeds – anything she wants.
- Keep her company while she breastfeeds.
- Be responsible for meal preparation and housework.
- Encourage her – breastfeeding two babies is a huge role. Tell her she's doing a fantastic job.

Sixteen bottles sitting on the bench

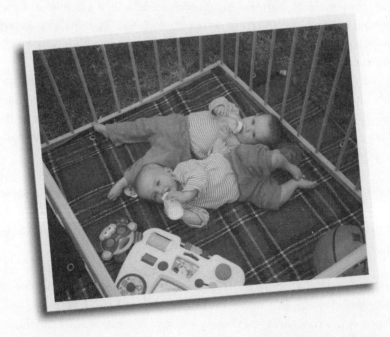

BOTTLE-FEEDING

BOTTLE-FEEDING: OUR STORIES

Many mothers bottle-feed their babies because they have tried unsuccessfully to breastfeed, while others choose to bottle-feed their twins from the beginning. There is evidence that the more informed parents are about bottle and breastfeeding before making a decision, the less likely they are to feel anxious or guilty about it.

If you intend to bottle-feed from day one, or intend to begin breastfeeding but change to bottle-feeding later, it's important to have information on hand to do it correctly and safely.

Katrina: When my babies were just over three months old, our maternal health nurse suggested that, because the girls had reflux and weren't gaining enough weight, it was time to put them on an anti-reflux formula. I wanted to continue to breastfeed so we compromised and decided to replace their four o'clock breastfeed with a bottle of anti-reflux formula.

We bought all the necessary equipment and offered the formula to the girls. Ella Hart drank her bottle, while Charlotte wouldn't have a bar of it. The next day I offered Charlotte expressed breastmilk in a bottle and she drank it happily. She continued to refuse formula but to drink expressed breastmilk so we tried a different brand of formula and after some cajoling were successful.

Giving the girls one bottle a day meant a proud dad, loving aunts, reluctant uncles, doting grandparents and best friends could help feed the babies. This made them all feel special and meant a break for me. If I was on my own for the bottle-feed, I could just prop the girls up on the pillows on my lap and hold the bottles.

The girls continued to have reflux until they were 12 months old, but overall their weights were improving and I'm sure that brief daily respite from feeding helped me re-charge and improve the quality of my supply for the rest of the night. One bottle a day meant we used a tin of anti-reflux formula a fortnight.

Louise: Fully bottle-feeding twins means making-up about 16 bottles of formula every day for two newborn babies. Three-hourly feeds at first, then after a couple of weeks four-hourly and it slowly cuts down from there.

The bottles are a fiddly business, but with all that practice you figure out a system fairly quickly. At first I boiled the bottles on the stove to sterilise them, standing with tongs and a huge saucepan of boiling water, splashing myself as I put them in and fished them out again. It was very time-consuming, I felt sad and poor ... then someone gave me a steam steriliser. After that I just washed the bottles, waited until there were six to sterilise, then popped them in the steam steriliser and turned it on. It did its own thing and turned itself off. I boiled the kettle and poured water into the sterilised bottles then put them into the fridge until I needed two. Then I'd pour the powder in and shake. To warm the milk before feeding the girls, I let the bottles sit and warm up in a jug of hot water.

I felt as though all I did for the first few months was make up formula and feed and change babies. I was envious of those who were fully breastfeeding both babies – sitting on a couch with your babies seemed so much more satisfying than running around organising bottles.

Whenever Celeste drank she got heartburn, causing her to be very unsettled and stopping her from feeding properly. She was finally diag-nosed with silent reflux. She wasn't vomiting often, which is why it is called 'silent', but would drink then suddenly stop and cry. She also did a funny licking movement with her tongue and lips which suggests reflux. The poor little thing had been having this painful burning in her digestive system all along. Reflux and silent reflux are quite common in pre-term and smaller babies.

Because the girls had been using bottles for so long I couldn't wait to move on to cups. The day they turned one I started them on cow's milk and by 14 months old they were only having one bottle. I cut that night-time bottle out by 18 months. If they had them much longer they'd want them forever, like their dummies. And they were drinking plenty of milk from cups.

Bottle-feeding with formula

There are advantages and disadvantages to consider when you're decid-ing how and what to feed your babies.

Some advantages of bottle-feeding with formula are:

- Formula-fed babies may not need to be fed as often as breastfed babies.
- Other people can mix the formula, sterilise and prepare the bottles and feed the babies, leaving you with some baby-free time.

ANOTHER MUM SAYS   'You have got to look after yourself, so you can look after the babies. So if it makes life easier to use formula, then do that.'

Some disadvantages of bottle-feeding with formula are:
- Formula-fed babies are more likely to have illnesses. Infections, eczema, wheezing, childhood diabetes and diarrhoea are also more common in formula-fed babies.
- Making up formula and sterilising equipment is a lot of work.
- Bottles, teats and formula cost money.

ANOTHER MUM SAYS   'For me, bottle-feeding was the best decision I could have made. Bottle-feeding meant my husband and others could help feed the babies, even in the middle of the night. When it was his turn to get up, I had no hesitation in rolling over and pushing him out of bed. Instead of just one or two hours straight sleep in the early days, I then got four or five hours sleep, which made an incredible difference to the way I felt the next day.'

ANOTHER MUM SAYS   'I started breastfeeding but one of my daughters wouldn't latch on properly and I needed to give her a bottle from early on. Bottle-feeding was so much easier for me because someone else could feed them as well.'

Infant formula

When buying your infant formula, check that it can be fed from birth. It should state this on the tin. Formulas that can be fed 'from birth' can be used from birth to 12 months. After 12 months babies can usually drink cow's milk, so there is no need to move on to a 'toddler' or 'follow-on' formula. There are also thickened formulas designed for babies with reflux, although there is no independent research showing these formulas are successful in their claims.

You can buy formula made from cow's milk, goat's milk or from soy liquid. Almost all soy formulas include genetically modified ingredients. You normally wouldn't use anything other than cow's milk formula unless for a medically diagnosed condition such as lactose intolerance. Check with your health practitioner before using any formula other than cow's milk formula.

It is fine to change your formula brand if you see a cheaper one or there are supply problems with your usual brand. All formula sold in Australia meets strict contents and quality guidelines. If you do switch, be careful to make up the formula according to the instructions on the tin as proportions vary with different brands. Too much formula for the amount of water can lead to a constipated baby or two, while not enough formula in the mix can lead to babies not gaining weight.

Making up formula safely

Making up bottles separately is the safest and most accurate way to prepare formula. It means less equipment, less chance of contamination and less chance of miscounting the number of scoops of formula.

- Empty the jug or kettle and refill it with water.
- Boil the water, then leave to cool.
- Wash your hands and set up on a clean bench or table.
- Pour the cooled boiled water into individual bottles.
- Using the scoop from inside the tin of formula, put the correct number of scoops into each bottle. Just scoop it in, don't push the formula in hard. Level the formula in the scoop with a knife.
- Pop the bottle disc and cap onto the bottle and shake gently.
- Store the bottles of formula on the back of the top shelf in the fridge, as the door shelves don't stay cold enough.
- Throw out any bottles of formula you haven't used within 24 hours.
- Throw out tins of formula that have been open for a month.
- Don't use formula past its 'use by' date.
- Warm the bottles for ten minutes or less.

You can save time by making up a quantity of formula in a jug, although it's not quite as accurate as making up individual bottles.

- Double-check the correct number of scoops needed for the water in your jug.
- Measure the correct number of scoops into a sterilised container and mark the level with permanent a marker. You can then use this container each time without having to risk losing count as long as you don't change formula brands.
- Measure the correct amount of cooled, boiled water into your measuring jug.

- Mix the formula with a sterilised spoon.
- Store the jug (covered) or the individual bottles in the coldest part of the fridge.

If you're going out and taking pre-mixed formula in bottles with you, they should be cold and kept in a cooler bag with an ice brick. Or you can take the boiled water and formula separately, then shake the formula in just before you feed the babies. This means it doesn't matter what temperature you keep the water.

> **ANOTHER MUM SAYS** 'We bought an urn and boiled a whole eight litres and made up all the bottles in the evening.'

Equipment

Bottles
You will need 8–12 large bottles.
- Before long, small bottles will be too small for your babies' increasing appetite, so save money and buy the larger ones from the start.
- There are no Australian standards on babies' bottles. There is a UK standard so if you buy bottles that meet them, they will be made of food-grade plastic and will be smooth on the inside. Smooth insides are important as crevices and spaces can harbour germs.
- Choosing clear rather than coloured or patterned bottles means you can see how clean they are.
- If you stick to the same brand, all the bits and pieces will fit together. All brands are much the same.
- Make sure your bottles are going to fit into the sterilising equipment you plan to use. Some steam sterilisers are designed for specific brands.

Teats
- Use one teat per bottle. A simple long, soft teat is probably best for newborn babies. Latex (rubber) is softer than silicone.
- As babies grow older you need to adjust the flow of the milk by increasing the number of holes in the teats.

> **A GENERAL GUIDE TO HOW MANY HOLES IN BOTTLE TEATS**
>
> 0–3 months = slow (one hole)
> 3–6 months = medium (two or three holes)
> 6–12 months = fast (three or four holes)

To check your babies' teats are giving a nice flow of milk, hold the bottle upside down. If the milk drips continuously your babies should be happy; if they need shaking or are flowing fast, change teats.

Babies drinking the thickened anti-reflux formulas will need a fast-flowing or cross-cut teat and the milk won't drip or flow out when you hold the bottle upside down, it will only come out if you squeeze.

Scoop

A scoop comes inside the tin. Don't use a scoop from a different brand tin as this could alter the strength of the formula. When you're measuring, you'll need a knife for levelling the formula in the scoop.

Bottlebrush

You'll need this to thoroughly clean bottles and teats.

Sterilising equipment

It's important to wash and sterilise bottles, teats and all the equipment used to make formula, as bits of milk can easily be trapped and breed bacteria which can make your babies sick. You need to keep sterilising bottles and teats until your babies are 12 months old.

The process involves:

- Rinsing everything in cold water straight after use.
- Washing everything in hot soapy water using a bottlebrush.
- Rinsing everything again.
- Sterilising everything.
- Refrigerating sterilised equipment for up to 24 hours until use.

STERILISING EQUIPMENT OPTIONS

- Buy or borrow a steamer. Microwave steam sterilisers or electric sterilisers are very quick and easy to use, they turn themselves off, don't cause fires and don't burn your fingers.
- Most dishwashers are also great for washing and sterilising bottles. Special containers are available to place teats, lids and all the bits into the dishwasher.
- You can sterilise on the top of the stove by boiling bottles and teats in a saucepan for five minutes. You will also need tongs to fish them out, a timer so you don't forget the bottles are on the stove, and a fire alarm and fire blanket just in case you do!
- Liquid sterilisers are also available where items soak in an anti-bacterial solution for at least one hour. These are chemically based and there is conflicting advice about whether or not to rinse items after sterilisation. The babies may taste the chemicals. The anti-bacterial solution can also kill healthy bacteria in the babies' gut. It can be a fiddly process because you also need to sterilise the tongs.

How to bottle-feed

You can heat bottles of formula by standing them in a container of hot or just boiled water for no longer than ten minutes as bacteria will start breeding at dangerous levels. The milk shouldn't be hot, just warm or body temperature. Test it by squirting a bit of your wrist, if it's too hot for the babies it will feel too hot on your wrist. Some babies are happy to drink cold formula and this is fine.

Heating bottles in a microwave isn't considered safe. Microwaves differ in their heating times so risk scalding babies' mouths. Microwaves cause hot spots to form in the milk so a bottle that seems warm can contain scalding hot spots. If you do use a microwave, shake the bottle vigorously and do the wrist temperature test.

You can prop them up in their rockers or using pillows while you hold their bottles. Use bottle-feeding as a chance to sit down with them, have a rest and share some happy feeding time.

- You can prop them in the 'underarm hold' twin feeding position (see page 151) so they are close to you on pillows in your lap while you hold their bottles.
- Or rest a head on each of your thighs or alongside each thigh.
- If your partner or a helper is available, it's lovely to feed a baby each, and have warm cuddles and eye contact.

Put the teats against your babies' lips and they should open their mouths and suck. Keep the teat of the bottle down so it is always filled with milk, so air bubbles don't get trapped and cause wind in your babies. To stop wind from building up, you can burp your babies if their sucking slows down mid-feed, as well as after the feed. If they go to sleep gently pop them on a shoulder and give them a back rub to wake them up before feeding again.

Your babies should take between 10 and 30 minutes to drink their bottles. Get slower teats if it takes them less than 10 minutes and faster teats for longer than 30. As your babies grow, they become much faster drinkers. Your babies may vary in their feeding times and amounts. This is normal for twins, just as it is for any babies of the same age.

The instructions on the tin of formula are an exact guide to preparing formula from that tin using that scoop, and a general guide to how much your babies will drink. If your babies are alert, have plenty of wet nappies and are gaining weight, then they're probably feeding well. If you have any doubts, talk to your doctor or maternal health nurse.

Putting your babies to bed with their bottles can cause problems with their teeth. Slow sucking in their sleep allows the milk to ferment in their mouths and causes tooth decay while their teeth are still forming. You can give them a dummy instead if they need to suck in bed.

(ANOTHER MUM SAYS) 'I don't heat bottles. They've had them cold or at room temperature from the start.'

Gastric Reflux

Gastric Reflux is a common term for Gastro-oesophical Reflux Disease (GORD). It's more frequent in babies born pre-term or with low birth weights.

It is normal for babies to lose a bit of milk when they're burped; it's also quite common for them to regurgitate large amounts. If one or both of your babies are regurgitating large amounts but are otherwise thriving and happy, then continue what you are doing: either formula or breastfeeding. Formula can be changed to a thickened 'reflux' formula as this may cut down the amount of regurgitation but there is no medical reason to use it. If you are concerned about your babies' regurgitation, constant screaming or feeding difficulties, consult your doctor. For more information on GORD see pages 189–190.

Combination feeding

Sometimes parents use a combination of breast and bottle-feeding. A bottle of either expressed breastmilk or formula can be given at alternate feeds or at certain times of the day.

Complementary feeds

Complementary feeds are bottle-feeds given to top up your breastfeed. If you are giving complementary formula feeds because you feel your supply is low, this will probably worsen the problem. As less milk is demanded by your babies, less will be produced.

However, there are times when babies are not gaining weight or are losing weight despite frequent feeding. 'Comping' with advice from a breastfeeding consultant will give you the best chance of continuing to breastfeed.

TO COMP FEED

- Breastfeed first.
- Try comping after the evening feed to start with.
- Offer the babies formula, as much or as little as they'd like.
- Express for 5–10 minutes, an hour after each feed, then store this breastmilk for later use.

If, with these strategies, you are unable to build up your supply, it is quite possible to feed a combination of breastmilk and formula for a long time.

Some parents of twins say that they were quite happy to fully breast-feed both babies but an occasional complement helped them get through a difficult period. This can be expressed breastmilk in a bottle or a formula feed.

ANOTHER MUM SAYS 'Early on I introduced a bottle as the last feed at night. I started with one and then introduced the second baby. Their weight gain hadn't been fantastic so both had this bottle-feed which helped them sleep. I'd had advice that if I start complementing with bottles my milk would dry up. I was breastfeeding twins, there was no way my milk was suddenly going to dry up.'

TIPS FOR SUCCESSFUL BOTTLE-FEEDING

- Have spare tins of formula in the cupboard.
- Borrow or buy a steam steriliser.
- Take a vacuum flask of boiling water if you need to warm bottles when you're out.
- Take a cold pack to keep milk cold if you're out for the day, or take formula and boiled water separately.
- Ask visitors to feed one baby while you feed the other.
- Breathe deeply and remember that you're doing a fantastic job.

TIPS FOR PARTNERS

- Support your partner's decision about her chosen form of feeding.
- Help to feed your babies as often as possible.
- Do some night feeds alone so you partner has some decent stretches of sleep.
- Take responsibility for sterilising bottles and preparing formula.

I'm completely alone except for two babies

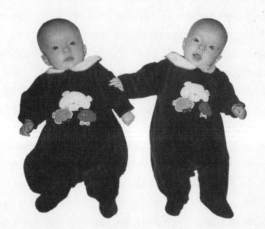

HOME

HOME: OUR STORIES

Parents who already have a child or two and are expecting twins start with some experience of babies, a relationship that has already adapted to having children, and some idea of what their new family may entail. They know the practical basics: how to hold and feed a baby and change nappies, so, although they may be busier, in some ways they have a head start. Their challenge is to move everyone over and make way for the new additions. Rearrange things. Be even busier. Adapt.

Those who haven't had children, or who suddenly find they have one or two babies who are more demanding than their others, may be shocked at what the reality of having twins involves. Your life with newborn twins may change everything in fundamental ways.

Katrina: Despite my apprehensions about managing with two babies, it was a relief and a joy to be home. Brad had the house spick-and-span and it was wonderful to breathe fresh air. The girls fell asleep in the car on the way home from hospital so we brought them inside without waking them. By the time we got the gear inside and set up the 'feeding station' the girls were ready for their feed. We were under paediatrician's orders to feed three-hourly. It took about an hour. Initially I set up on the couch in the spare room, thinking that it would be nice to have privacy when we had visitors. In reality I found this very isolating and the visitors usually ended up sitting in the spare room with me, so I just moved to the lounge and gave up being embarrassed about 'baring all'.

My mum and Brad looked after the house, the washing and meals. I was busy looking after the babies and getting some sleep but their help meant I could have a free hand to write the thank you letters, time to chat with visitors and an opportunity to recover. I was expecting this to be the worst time of my life but it was actually quite civilised. I was waiting for the hard part. I know it was all reasonably pleasant because there were three of us focusing on keeping the babies happy and the house in order. Three of us made those first six weeks manageable and enjoyable.

From the start we were out and about. The day after our arrival home, Mum and I popped out to the shops leaving the girls alone with their father. This was two weeks after the caesar but I was able to drive and felt full of energy. I was out for an hour and a half in total but I felt incredibly liberated. I also felt a bit incomplete.

The girls had various appointments in those first weeks, so we were forced out the door. Up to the hospital to have Charlotte's harness fitted. Off to the Multiple Birth Association playgroup, to weekly sessions at the physio, or to the hospital for ultrasounds of the girls' hips. There were new parents' group, shopping trips to town and more doctor's visits. We also had visitors and made some social visits ourselves. Our days were very full. We were rarely out of the house longer than two hours because I would try to be home for feeds. I was feeding them together so I didn't want to risk our three-hourly routine.

Having twins meant we were entitled to home visits from the maternal health nurse, rather than going to the clinic. We kept up this arrangement for seven months. We had so many outings that it was easier to have a home-based appointment. There was so little time between feeds.

The visiting nurses were a wonderful resource and crucial in helping us through the first year. Not only did they monitor the girls' weight gains and developmental milestones but they were there to help me. I constantly discussed sleeping and feeding issues with them and they were always ready to listen and source of advice. I was able to discuss with them my fears and feelings of inadequacy. They would reassure me that I was doing a great job. They were surprised I'd managed to continue breastfeeding twins and recognised that I was well organised and able to get out and socialise.

My mother was invaluable. Not only her domestic help but just watching her talk and soothe the babies, helped give me ideas on how to do it. She also helped me feel relaxed and that it's OK to do my own thing with them. I was constantly caught up in the how I 'should' be doing it and referring to the literature, whereas my mother gave me permission to do what *I* felt was right. Not once did she tell me what to do or how, she let me find my own way. I had to ask her when I wanted her advice.

I had the energy through the day to feed and look after the girls, but I didn't have energy for much else. Interrupted sleep and night feeds were physically exhausting and I tried to sleep nearly each time the girls did. I generally managed eight hours sleep during a 24-hour period. I only managed this because of my mother and husband. I rarely had the time or energy to talk on the phone or even to watch TV. I would have dinner and go to bed.

Breastfeeding, carrying and changing babies were causing pains in my neck and shoulders. After being home two weeks it was almost unbearable and I booked in for a massage. The massage was therapeutic and released a lot of tension. It also motivated me to improve my posture while feeding to reduce the strain on these muscles. I would try to look straight ahead rather than down at my babies which put my neck and shoulders at such a crooked angle.

A huge part of me was very happy. I had two beautiful girls, we were all doing well and it wasn't as hard as I thought it would be. Another part of me was absolutely underwhelmed. Parenthood was a real anticlimax. I was expecting to feel fulfilled. I felt just the same old me on the inside, except now I was suddenly a mother, but I didn't really know what that meant yet.

Louise: Finally … bringing home the newborn babies.

Tony was working that day and didn't get paid if he didn't turn up, no matter what the excuse. We needed the money so he went to work. I arranged for my sister-in-law to collect the babies and me from hospital in my car with the two capsules fitted.

We did a chemist stop on the way and opened an account. I panic-bought bottles, formula, bottom creams, dummies and far too much unnecessary stuff. Then home to a spotless house. Classical music playing softly. I felt surprisingly calm and very happy. My sister-in-law had to leave to pick up her kids so I was left completely alone.

Except for two babies.

Three-hourly feeds took about an hour, breastfeeding both girls – usually simultaneous feeding, then topping both up with formula. This left two hours in between for nappy changing, eating, housework, sleeping and entertaining visitors.

My 'sign on the door' mentality that I'd relied on in hospital was short-lived. Without the nursing staff, I lost my commitment to being selfish and sensible. I was determined in those very early days to appear as though I was coping well. I wanted people to look at me and say how well I was doing with two babies. This meant that I let anyone who rang come by for a look and pretended I was fine, even if I was exhausted. I insisted on making the coffee or lunch and didn't complain about a thing. I let people stay for as long as they liked and probably encouraged them to stay longer. I felt it would be rude to put a 'No Visitors' sign on the door. Somehow I felt it was my duty to share these babies with everyone who'd been so interested and so generous during my pregnancy.

I had no routine, not because I chose to, but because I didn't know what a routine was. I imagined a pattern would emerge, that the babies would fall asleep when they were tired and would let me know when they were hungry, and I'd change their nappies a lot. They didn't fall asleep when they were tired and I couldn't tell when they were tired. Or hungry. It was chaotic but I kept insisting that everything was fine.

In my determination to be superhuman, I insisted on Tony and I walking the girls to their five-week maternal and child health clinic check-up, about an hour each way. We popped the babies in the pram and headed off on our very long walk. At the health centre they were both weighed, measured and found to be doing fine.

Celeste was unhappy on the way there and completely beside herself screaming on the way home. We stopped to pop her dummy back in and try to comfort her many times but it seemed to make no difference, so we decided to charge on home, well aware that such a long walk had been a big mistake. We had no option but to walk all the way home, as we couldn't easily catch a cab or a bus with the double pram and two babies.

About ten minutes from home we were marching along the footpath full steam ahead, hurrying home because the baby wouldn't stop howling. We stopped at the road to cross. No cars coming.

'Oh look, someone's dropped their doll on the road.' I stepped over it and kept walking, then turned around as the horror dawned on me. 'Oh my god, that's my baby!' I ran back and picked her up, leaving Tony and Camille where they stood and charged into the doctor's. Thankfully, we were almost outside the medical clinic.

The doctor saw us immediately and checked Celeste thoroughly and assured me that she was absolutely fine. No bleeding, no bruises, no sign in fact that she'd hit the road.

The shock didn't set in until later that night. Always use the harnesses no matter how young the baby. Celeste had pushed herself backwards using her feet and fallen into the elasticised underside of the pram, then rolled out onto the road. I still dream of cars coming around that corner.

In retrospect, I think planning how life will work at home before you arrive is extremely important. We had a 'wait and see what feels right' approach to coming home. Unusual for me, a list writer, planner and highly organised person. I had spent almost no time around newborns. Certainly not enough time to notice that mothers had routines, that babies needed to be put to bed rather than just falling asleep wherever they were. I was completely winging it, without a clue.

Daily life

Daily life with two babies can be more manageable with some help, routines, the right company and some short cuts.

Newborn routine

Babies like routine and thrive on reasonable regularity. The newborn routine is a continuous link of change-feed-play-sleep. Newborns are usually awake to be changed, fed, and cuddled then are back to bed.

Routine from 3–6 months.

Some families are quite happy going with the flow with no routine. Others are happier if they at least have a plan for how the day will go. The following is a flexible guide we have adapted to suit two babies.

5 a.m. to 8 a.m.	Babies wake, breastfeed or bottle. Stay up for about an hour. Maybe bath. Put to sleep – may sleep half an hour to two hours
9 a.m. to 12 noon	Breastfeed or bottle, plus food from a spoon if appropriate. Up for about an hour. Put to sleep or go out. Baby may sleep half an hour to two hours
1 p.m. to 4 p.m.	Breastfeed or bottle, plus food from a spoon if appropriate. Babies may only sleep for a short period. Awake the remainder of the time. This may be a whingy, grizzly part of the day. Go for a walk.
5 p.m. to 7 p.m.	Maybe bath. Breastfeed or bottle and/or other food if appropriate. Avoid letting your babies have a late catnap, if you can, as this can interfere with bedtime.
7 p.m. to 8 p.m.	Bedtime. Try to keep bedtime regular and consistent no matter what happens during the rest of the day. Total sleeping in the day varies from one to four hours and can vary between babies. A number of babies only catnap. It is usually very difficult to make babies who catnap during the day sleep more or longer.

If your babies have the same routine each day they may be more settled, as they'll know what to expect. If they are always put to sleep in the same way, they'll probably respond to the consistency.

ANOTHER MUM SAYS 'I kept accidentally banging their heads on door frames as I got used to navigating my way around carrying two babies.'

Bathing

Two babies can make for a juggling act at bath time. Through trial and error you'll find a bathing routine that suits you, but initially it can be exhausting work. Newborn babies don't need to be bathed every day. They usually get a good wipe at nappy change time and you can wipe their hands and faces in between times. Even older babies suffer no harm if they miss a bath now and then. Some parents bath one baby a night so the babies have a bath on alternate nights.

Others can't bear the thought of bathing only one when it's not much more effort to bath the second while everything is handy. And bathing babies before bed, then putting them in clean fresh pyjamas may help them settle.

If it's just you at bath time, have both babies in the room with you. Have everything ready before you start – towels, wash cloths, baby wash, clothes, nappies and nappy rash cream. You may be using the baby bath, the laundry tub or the big bath. Your babies will be happier if the room is warm. Undress and bathe one baby at a time, putting the other in a rocker or near some toys while waiting their turn.

You might even choose to bathe with them, but you'd generally need another pair of hands around to do this. Another option is to pop one at a time in the shower with a parent. Wet babies get very slippery though and this can feel quite dangerous. Some babies love the shower, others don't.

ANOTHER MUM SAYS 'I found bathing them a very exhausting process. We had a sunken bath which was impossible so we'd set up the whole bathing station in the kitchen. Before they could crawl, we'd usually only bathe them every second or third night and they'd get a wipe with a warm flannel in between.'

Help at home

Often the best help when your two newborns arrive is with practical things like cooking, cleaning, washing and shopping. This gives you time to get to know and learn how to care for your babies. If others can help keep the household together, you can focus on yourself and your babies.

Once visitors arrive and have admired your babies, you can ask them to hang the washing on the line, make you a coffee or peel some potatoes. If you find it hard to ask people for help, you could have a tick list of jobs and when people casually ask if there's anything they can do, you can equally casually reply, 'There's a list on the fridge'.

Parents of twins are often inundated with offers of help which may or may not translate into actual help. 'Help' can be a double-edged sword. While an extra pair of hands is always useful, sometimes it also means someone in the way. Many parents find they need to follow-up on the offers with those they would like and schedule in the help.

ANOTHER MUM SAYS   'Although it's hard to admit, I often found the days my husband was home and wanting to help more with the babies were a lot harder for me. It meant I had to incorporate him into the equation and work in with his needs. I found not only did I have to deal with two screaming babies but that I had to liaise, negotiate and compromise with him as to how we were going to deal with them. When it was just me, I could get on with it my way.'

Organising your time

- For the first couple of weeks, if possible, make feeding the babies your only job.
- If you can afford it, pay someone to clean your house. If you can't afford it, suggest someone offer you cleaning as a present.
- Think about organising friends and family to help on a roster system. When someone comes to visit, give them a job to do.
- Prioritise. Put up a list of what really needs doing. Plan ahead – the evening hours are often the most stressful, so think about preparing dinner in the morning. If the house looks beautiful but you're exhausted then re-prioritise.
- Encourage people to ring before they turn up so they can pick up milk, bread, or whatever you need.

- Talk with other new mums of twins to share information and ideas. If you're not in contact already call the new parent contact at your local AMBA and ask to be put in contact with one or two others. Don't be afraid to ring. They understand. Or pack up the family and turn up at an AMBA playgroup. You can ask advice from those who've been there and there will be plenty of nostalgic mums to cuddle your babies.
- Let the answering machine answer the phone. Call back when you're ready.
- Leave the house every day, even if it's only for a few minutes.
- Organise some time alone.
- Set up an account with a pharmacy and a supermarket that home-delivers (most do).
- Eat widely and wisely but don't panic if it's not three full meals a day. Takeaways and frozen dinners will keep you going for a while. Eat healthy snacks like fruit, yoghurt, wholemeal rolls, roast chicken, cheese and hommus.
- Just an extra pair of hands at any time will usually be useful. If friends and family aren't available think about other contacts like the local TAFE childcare students, teenage or adult neighbour, helpers through the local church, volunteers through your local council or your maternal and child care nurse may have other suggestions.
- If you don't have a good support network, ask AMBA or NZMBA for help.

ANOTHER MUM SAYS   'I did not allow any help for a long time. When we did arrange a paid carer, I stayed with her. I learnt the hard way that you need to get someone to help as soon as you can, even if you do stay at home with them.'

ANOTHER MUM SAYS   'I get a break when I ask for one. I play netball one night a week. My partner is happy to look after the girls and I can go shopping, read a book or visit a friend. It's a necessity. Initially I tried to have time-out when the babies were sleeping to make it easier for him. Now it's whenever I feel like it.'

Six-week check-up

See your GP or obstetrician six to eight weeks following the birth of your babies for a general examination of your physical and mental health. The doctor will check your breasts, uterus and cervix. If it's over 12 months since your last Pap smear, this might be a good time to have one. This is also a good opportunity to talk about how you are feeling and to organise a referral to an expert, if necessary.

What do I do with crying babies?

It's quite normal for newborns to be unsettled for four hours or more each day and on at least one day each week. Thirty seconds of babies' crying can sometimes feel like an hour. Babies usually cry for a reason. It is their way of communicating. They're not trying to annoy you, they're trying to get their needs met. Crying is an important part of babies' natural development and helps them release tension. It can also be a great cause of tension for parents.

Your babies could be crying because:
- they are hungry
- they need a nappy change
- they are tired or overtired
- they want social stimulation
- they are over stimulated (too much eye contact, too many cuddles, lots of activity)
- they are unwell
- they are too hot or cold
- they are in pain.

When crying, babies can squirm and seem uncomfortable. They may turn red and draw up their legs as though in pain. Often this is described as 'wind' but this is rarely why babies are crying. If they're pushing their arms and legs this is part of their crying and can mean they're over stimulated and ready to rest.

By about three months of age babies usually cry less. They learn to cope with the things going on around them and develop other ways of communicating like smiling and making sounds. They also become interested in new activities like watching and sucking their hands.

Two crying babies

ANOTHER MUM SAYS   'When they both cried, I did too.'

Often with twins one baby is more unsettled than the other. They can also swap roles, but you may still find you're usually only settling one crying baby at a time. The times when both babies are upset can be very stressful and difficult to manage, especially if you are alone. Handling two babies can be very difficult if you are trying to calm one baby and the other is screaming. Parents of twins can get distressed at these times, but you can only do your best.

Sometimes your efforts to stop their crying may not help and the babies become over stimulated. If your efforts haven't worked within 15 minutes then they probably won't work. Before you get too frazzled, you could try putting the babies down in a quiet place and leaving them to it for five minutes. They may be happy just to have some peace and you may appreciate a break from the crying. If you take a few deep breaths, have a cuppa, phone a friend or do something else for a little while, you may feel ready to try settling them again. If you decide to let them cry it out, check them every five minutes to make sure they're OK. If they seem to have gone to sleep, check they're OK and leave them in peace.

ANOTHER MUM SAYS   'There were times when I'd just let them scream. They were comfortable and fed and safe in their rockers. I was exhausted, emotionally more than anything. I felt there was nothing more I could do for them, so I went down and laid on my bed. When I rejoined them and picked them up for a cuddle they cheered up and I was refreshed and able to cope again.'

Learn how to keep yourself calm when you are getting upset because your babies are crying. The calmer you are, the better able you will be to soothe your babies. Persist – the time will pass. Choose ways of dealing with unpleasant or difficult situations. You could try:

- Deep breathing.
- Thinking about all the good aspects of having children.
- Remembering that the current situation won't last forever.
- Accepting it's hard and using your knowledge and skills to deal with it.

TIPS TO CALM A CRYING BABY

- Make sure each of your babies is dressed comfortably and their room is at around 17–20 degrees Celsius. If their hands or feet are cold or warm it doesn't mean they are uncomfortable. Check that their tummies, backs and the back of their necks are warm rather than cold or hot and clammy.
- Change your baby's nappy. A wet disposable nappy shouldn't make a baby cry.
- Tiredness is a common cause of whingeing and crying. Classic tiredness signs include yawning, grizzling, jerky movements of arms and legs and crying.
- Babies who have become overtired can have problems falling asleep and staying asleep.
- If your baby is gaining weight and has regular wet nappies (6–8 per day), then the crying is unlikely to be caused by hunger or thirst. It could be an appetite increase though, and these usually last one or two days.
- If you are breastfeeding, you could try feeding each baby more often to comfort them. Formula-fed babies shouldn't be given extra feeds unless they need extra food.
- Put something by their cots that smells of you – it could be something you've been wearing that day.
- Cuddle and soothe them. Hold the babies upright close to your body and hum.
- Try giving them a dummy.
- Move with your babies around the house or take them outside. Slings or pouches may help. Their screaming is never as loud outside.
- Put them in the pram and rock it gently or take them for a walk.
- Bathe or massage them.
- Use music – either with a definite beat or relaxation music.
- Sometimes sounds such as a vacuum cleaner or exhaust fan can make babies sleepy.

Colic

About one quarter of babies are reported to experience 'colic'. There are a variety of definitions of colic. It is not a disease or condition, but more a description for a regularly upset baby who can cry for hours each day. Causes are not known but colic is often incorrectly attributed to wind pain or allergies. The good news is that babies grow out of it usually by the time they are about three months old.

Gastro-oesophical Reflux Disease (GORD)

Reflux is the back flow of food from the stomach into the gullet, usually after meals. It happens in humans of all ages, not just babies, and is not usually noticed as the oesophageal sphincter, or muscle at the top of the stomach, works to keep the food down where it's supposed to be.

Diagnoses of Gastro-oesophical Reflux Disease are very difficult as the symptoms are behavioural: screaming, back arching and drink refusal. These symptoms could either be GORD or another reason for an 'unsettled' baby.

Gastro-oesophical Reflux Disease can cause a small number of usually pre-term or sick babies to regurgitate then draw some of the contents of their stomach into the lungs causing wheezing coughing, wheezing, breathing difficulties or pneumonia. A specialist doctor is needed for the care of these babies.

Gastro-oesophical Reflux Disease can cause pain or heartburn in some babies making them averse to drinking. These babies, if they aren't drinking enough, will lose weight and not thrive so they need a specialist doctor.

Unsettled crying babies are often over diagnosed and treated for acid reflux. Occasionally, though, acid reflux is a problem and can be so severe that the gullet becomes ulcerated and the baby vomits blood. This also needs immediate treatment from a specialist doctor.

To treat a baby with suspected Gastro-oesophical Reflux Disease sleep her so her head is uphill and try to feed her in this tilted position. If a baby has acid reflux numerous short feeds are usually more easily tolerated than less frequent long feeds. Many health professionals are reluctant to diagnose acid reflux too hastily but acknowledge that it does affect some babies and will prescribe medication once they are convinced a baby is suffering from this rare condition.

ANOTHER MUM SAYS 'One of my babies was having about nine feeds a day, vomiting half of each feed then crying. I tried everything I could think of to keep him happy. I tried giving him a bottle but he just scoffed it and vomited, he vomited less when breastfeeding because he had to work harder to get the milk so it slowed him down. My doctor finally understood the problem when my baby threw up all over his room.'

ANOTHER MUM SAYS 'I knew something was wrong with my baby because she would start to feed then after five minutes suddenly stop and scream. It was always at exactly the same time during every feed. When someone suggested what it was I had to wait a couple of days for her Zantac (medication) to kick in. The Zantac worked brilliantly for a couple of months then when the problem started again I realised she'd grown and needed a bigger dose. She took it for about six months then I slowly weaned her off and the problem was gone.'

Immunisations

This is doubly important with twins – if you forget both, they tend to catch things from each other, and a bout of illness can be drawn out for weeks.

If your babies came early it is recommended that you go by their actual age rather than using their corrected age for immunisations. Immunisations are no different with twins except that after the needle two at a time can be difficult to comfort. You can take them to separate appointments or, ideally, take someone else with you so you can each comfort a baby. It is often suggested that giving your babies the recommended dose of paracetamol prior to the injection can help reduce and control pain and fever secondary to immunisation.

ANOTHER MUM SAYS 'When my twins contracted chickenpox I was solely breastfeeding them. Each of my three children got chickenpox two weeks apart and we were in quarantine for six weeks. I'd highly recommend the vaccine that is now available, as I wouldn't wish our stressful experience on anyone.'

Unwell babies

A baby's average body temperature is 37 degrees Celsius. A baby under three months old with a raised temperature (above 37.5 degrees) should be taken to see a doctor, unless the baby has just been immunised so the cause of the fever is known and it will run its course and disappear.

Babies aged three to twelve months should see a doctor if their temperature is above 40 degrees. If their temperature is between 37.5 and 39 degrees but they are otherwise happy and comfortable that don't necessarily need to see a doctor.

If your baby is hot and irritable undress her to a singlet and nappy and give her a dose of paracetamol or ibuprofen. Give her extra fluids and see your doctor if the fever doesn't clear up or if you are troubled.

IF ANY OF THESE SYMPTOMS OCCUR CONTACT YOUR DOCTOR AS SOON AS POSSIBLE

- Fever or chill – a temperature below 36.5 degrees or above 37.2 degrees for over 24 hours
- Vomiting large amounts over a 24-hour period or longer
- Vomiting green bile
- Spots or a rash
- Lethargy, sluggishness or a lack of interest in feeding when the baby is normally quite alert
- Decrease in the wetness of nappies
- Blood in their poo or vomit
- Swelling in the belly
- Waking up over and over in the night screaming with pain

Getting out and about

At first, your life will probably be easier if people can come to you. In the early months, life revolves around sleeping and feeding and, while it's hard to fit in travelling and visiting, sometimes it's worth the effort. It can be lovely when your babies are young and will lie, sit or sleep in their pram.

ANOTHER MUM SAYS 'I hardly ever left the house, only for doctor's appointments. It was just so difficult to pack up and get out. It could get quite lonely but I saw my parents almost every day. Some days I'd be in tears and ring Mum, who'd say, 'Put everyone in the car and come over.' Then I could have a shower in peace, there were three pairs of hands to look after the three kids.'

ANOTHER MUM SAYS When my boys were twelve months old, I separated from their father. Up until then, I'd been able to leave the babies at home with him and go out. Then suddenly I had to completely change the way I lived, socially. I had very little money and couldn't afford babysitters whenever I wanted them and there are only so many times you can dump twins on friends and family!
So I became someone who rarely went out, but I made a real effort to have an open-house policy so that anyone could drop in at any time of the day or evening. I made myself invite people over even if I didn't really feel like it – if I hadn't made that effort, I would have been completely alone except for two babies, and I would have slowly gone mad. Friends who didn't have kids came over after the boys had gone to bed, around 8 pm. More often than not they would bring dinner and always a bottle of wine which meant I could be my old self for a few hours. People who had children came round during the day so we could wear out all the kids down at the park, and then I'd make a slap-up dinner for all of us.
I was still lonely in a relationship sense because I was the sole parent of two extremely active and demanding boys, but I didn't feel trapped or stuck at home on my own because it was too hard to go out. I couldn't go out into the world so I made sure the world came to me. And the best part of all is that those early years formed the basis of many long-standing friendships and the boys became very social too, because we always had people around us.'

What to pack on an outing

If you take two newborns out, you should get by with:

- four nappies
- two changes of clothing
- change mat
- nappy wipes (which you can also use to 'wash' your hands)
- nappy rash cream or powder
- spare bibs
- two cloth nappies to dry their bottoms and mop up spills
- plastic bags for dirty nappies and clothes
- any medication your babies may need
- bottles with water and formula if bottle feeding
- depending on the weather, baby rugs, hats and pram weather shields
- water bottle and snacks for you.

TIPS FOR GETTING OUT IN THE EARLY DAYS

- Practise setting up and folding down your twin pram before you think about leaving the house.
- Keep your keys, phone and bag in the same place so you can get out more quickly.
- Have your nappy bag packed and ready the night before so it's not a rush to get it all together. When you come home from outings, re-stock the bag so it's ready next time you go out.
- Shower the night before and have your clothes chosen and ready to wear.
- Plan where you're going and how you're going to get there. Allow lots of time so you don't feel rushed.
- Get someone to come with you. An extra pair of hands or moral support can be a big help during those early outings.
- If going out to appointments, phone in advance to check they're running on time. If you're running late, that's OK, just ring and let them know.
- Load the car first, babies last – don't put your babies down on the driveway.
- Be careful where you park the stroller while you unload babies from the car and always put the brake on.

Attention when you're out

Some parents enjoy the attention that their twins attract, while others would prefer to do without it. Often it depends on how you're feeling that day and how much time you have. You may decide to limit conversation to other parents of multiples, as they'll be out there too! You will feel instantly bonded and usually have tips to share.

TO AVOID ATTENTION

- Smile confidently and keep walking.
- Dress babies differently and carry one in a pouch and one in the stroller, then there's less chance they'll be identified as twins.
- Put the sunshade over the babies' pram so they can still see out but others can't see in.

FAMOUS PARENTS OF TWINS:

- William Shakespeare fathered boy/girl twins
- Kerry Armstrong (Australian actor best known for her roles in 'Seachange' and 'Lantana') has twin boys
- Ingrid Bergman (actor) and Roberto Rossellini (director) had twins, Isabella Rossellini was one of the pair
- Roberto De Niro (actor) had twins
- Michael J Fox (actor) has boy/girl twins
- Bing Crosby (actor and singer)
- Muhammad Ali (boxer)
- Mia Farrow (actor) and Andre Previn (musician and conductor)
- Loretta Lynn (country and western singer) has twin daughters
- Ricky Nelson (musician)
- Pele (soccer legend)
- Denzel Washington (actor)
- Mel Gibson (actor)
- President George W. Bush (President of USA) and wife, Laura, have twin daughters
- Margaret Thatcher (former British Prime Minister) and husband, Denis
- Ernie Sigley (radio personality)
- Al Pacino (actor) and Beverley D'Angelo (actor)
- Julia Roberts (actor)
- Ben Elton (author and comedian)

Some mothers find it's more trouble than it's worth or too time-consuming to take the babies out and prefer to go out at times when someone else can look after them.

> (ANOTHER MUM SAYS) 'Some days I needed to make an extra effort to motivate myself to go to the local park to see other mums and get some sunshine and fresh air. It's always worth it though, it was a break from the babies and time-out for me.'

Feeling very busy

Coming home with your new babies can alter every aspect of your life. You may be learning to do many things you've never done before and be feeling tired and very busy. Adjusting to your new life may make you feel confused or depressed.

> (ANOTHER MUM SAYS) 'Time-saving strategies for me have included changing and dressing the twins as soon as they wake in the morning; always having dinner cooked before my son comes home from school; and the older boys often having a shower at night with their dad. I think it's good to get babies in the shower early from when they're young. 'It's hell in this house between 6 and 8 p.m. We let the answering machine take messages during the night which really lifts the stress and helps us keep some control and helps our relationship with each other. The most important people are at home, the rest of the world can wait till the morning or at least till the kids are all asleep.'

Work out what is important. List the main things that *need* to get done and then the things that you *want* to get done. Cross off as you go. If you put the list somewhere visible, your partner or helpers can complete and cross off things as they go.

If you are concerned that you are doing too much, look after your own family first. Think about what you do and don't want to do, and practise saying 'no' nicely. Make it a family policy to accept all genuine offers of help, food and baby-sitting. Operate remotely as much as possible – Medicare claims by mail, banking on line . . .

ANOTHER MUM SAYS   'I only do things that are absolutely necessary. At the start of the day my main priority is to have a shower, get dressed and put on my lipstick. I'd rather put my make-up on than do the dishes. I do all my shopping online or over the phone. If I've got half an hour to spare I'd rather go and have a coffee than go to the supermarket.'

Getting it together

During those early days at home, keep in mind that no one is an expert – we all just have ideas that may or may not work. Parenthood can be a very hard job and we do learn as we go. There are good times and bad times but most days are a combination of both. A break helps you to have the energy to keep going. And most importantly, enormous support comes from contact with other parents of twins.

ANOTHER MUM SAYS   'Now closer to two in age, our girls are a huge source of pride and joy. Our confidence has grown along with our patience. We laugh with them most of the time and shout occasionally. Most importantly, we've forgiven ourselves for any misdemeanours and we know our children feel loved by us, as do we by them.'

TIPS FOR SURVIVING BEING ALONE WITH TWO BABIES

- Make yourself remember that this super-intensive high-demand phase will not last forever.
- Write a list of positive things about yourself, your partner and your babies. Think about your plans and goals for your family.
- Remember that there aren't any hard and fast rules for what works – do what suits you and your family.
- Accept genuine offers of help and learn to say 'No thanks' nicely when it doesn't feel right.
- If you can afford it, consider paying for help around the house.
- Contact other families with twins for shared understanding.

TIPS FOR PARTNERS

- If you're at work during the day, make sure you're involved with the babies in the early mornings and evenings. Remember that she's been alone with them all day.
- Make time to do something special when the babies are asleep at night.
- Stay calm when she's upset, even though you're tired too. Hold your tongue when required and find a way that works to support your partner and children in difficult moments.
- Be helpful rather than critical. If things aren't going too well, choose a time when you feel calm to discuss a new approach for the whole family.
- Give her a hug and tell her she's wonderful and that you and the babies are lucky to have her.
- Let her know that you consider looking after two babies is a team effort and that you're on the same team.

Bert Newton is my new best friend

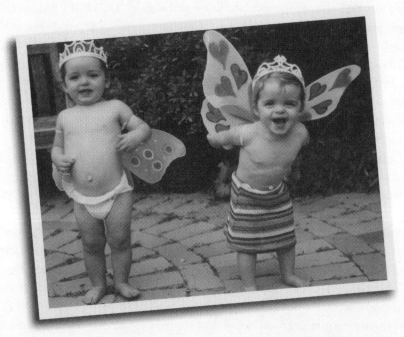

MOTHERHOOD

MOTHERHOOD: OUR STORIES

Motherhood is full of contradictions. At times your day can be very peaceful then suddenly it's really rowdy. Mothers often experience moments of pure love and adoration then moments of pure frustration. Some mothers feel their day is mundane and their achievements are small. We can feel as though there's nothing to talk about beyond how much our babies fed and slept today. With two new babies, sometimes it seems that as soon as one baby is happy, the other suddenly becomes miserable.

Katrina: If I had to use one word to describe motherhood, it would have been 'breastfeeding'. I was quite confused. I thought children were going to enhance my full life. I was learning a lot – how to breastfeed, how to function one-handed, how little resistance I had to crying babies – but nothing terribly rewarding. I felt unsatisfied. Nothing met my expectations. I was no longer living a full and complete life. I was just a mother now and it wasn't enough.

My feelings about motherhood were ambivalent. I loved my babies but I also resented what their arrival had done to my life. I started devising all sorts of ways of getting rid of them. Suddenly my death looked like a good option. I'd rather die than have to deal with all this feeding, cleaning, settling, and trying to sleep. I fantasised about running away. I had a passport and a credit card. I could disappear and start again. All this crazy stuff went through my mind. But it really helped me to know that I always had other options. I didn't have to stay, I was choosing to stay.

I thought I'd made a terrible mistake. I thought my relationship with Brad was in danger. I was angry at myself for going into parenthood with so little idea of what it would be like. I hadn't done my research. When I planned a baby, I felt I would be making my life complete. Instead, it seemed I existed solely to feed, clothe and clean up after them. I was meeting this purpose – but why? Who could want this dull existence? Why didn't other mothers tell me it would be like this? I had ambitions beyond being a cook, cleaner and nursemaid – but as a mother, these were my new jobs.

My husband was doing so much but I continued to be very unhappy, to regret that I had ever decided to have children. One day he said he just wanted me to be happy, he would look after the girls and I could leave.

We cried and cried. I knew I could never go through with it. I could never leave my babies and look at myself in the mirror again.

Many times I continued to wish I had only one baby. Two were really hard work. One would be crying while her sister was being attended to. All this crying that mothers of one don't have to endure. All this crying my babies shouldn't have to endure – it's not fair on them that they have to wait for their sister all the time. I thought they might learn to be patient. They never did. I tried very hard to focus on the good things but at times I would get down again and it was hard to see beyond the 'bad'. They were such good girls, sleeping and feeding relatively well, yet I still felt it was awful.

Some conjoined twins were born in Brisbane – joined at the head. So many things reminded me how lucky I *should* feel. I had everything I had ever wanted – a wonderful husband and two healthy and beautiful daughters – yet I was still unhappy.

About five months in, I reached a point where I knew I needed some professional counselling. I was smiling on the outside and getting on with life but I was full of anger and resentment. I started to break things – throwing glasses across the room. I felt out of control. I didn't think I would hurt my babies, although part of me wanted to. I thought I was more likely to hurt myself or my husband. The maternal nurse was the first person I asked for a referral and she was able to put me onto the local Community Health Centre which had a counselling service available, funded by the public health system. The counselling was difficult but fantastic. I had an initial appointment where I was 'assessed' and judged a high priority case. This shocked me. Surely there were nutters out there who were *really* going to kill someone who should be the priority, but I was grateful this meant I would get help soon.

I felt self-conscious hanging about in the waiting room before my appointment. Did being here mean I was mentally ill? Am I really a legitimate case? At the same time I was proud of myself for seeking help. During part of my first session I filled out a brief questionnaire designed to help diagnose postnatal depression. Apparently I had a moderate case. The counsellor recommended I talk to my GP about antidepressants. I was reluctant. I felt angry but I really felt I had good reason to be angry. I didn't think my feelings were caused by some chemical imbalance. I wasn't just ungrateful. People struggle with one baby. I had two. I was also very angry with other mothers. Why didn't they tell me it would be like this? Why do they keep the reality a secret? Why does everyone congratulate you when you're going to have a baby when they could be more helpful by being more honest about their experiences. Most of all, I was angry with myself. Why the hell did I go into this parenthood caper so ill-prepared?

I felt if I started on drugs now, the problems I had would never be resolved. I was told that many new mums take them for a while and it helps them get over a rough patch so they're better able to deal with their lives. Later when they have more strength, they can stop taking them. I didn't completely rule out the possibility. I felt it was an option if counselling didn't work for me.

My counsellor was wonderful and I was able to be incredibly honest about my feelings. I was able to say things to her that I couldn't say to anyone else. She also asked the right questions. Counselling helped put me back in control. I saw her twice the first month and then another two times over a couple of months. I just made another appointment when I felt I needed to. It helped keep me going. It helped me understand myself and what I wanted and how parenthood hadn't lived up to my expectations. I loved my children but I didn't enjoy being with them all the time. Counselling helped me accept that and move on, instead of resenting my children or being angry at myself because of it. It also helped me identify what I needed to make things better for us – childcare!

When the girls were 11 months old they started childcare three days a week. They loved it and it was a turning point for us all.

Louise: When I was young I had a sister who died of SIDS. The more tired I became, the more convinced I was that something was going to go terribly wrong. I heard a radio interview with a woman who argued that SIDS had a genetic link. After hearing this I felt I had to watch the babies most of the night to check that they were breathing. Of course I'd hop back into bed knowing they had been breathing a minute ago but had to get up again straightaway to make sure they still were. Up, down, up, down – anxious, exhausted mother.

I started to get very sleep-deprived fairly quickly and resented the fact that the girls were sleeping in our room. My only time for potential peace, space and rest had BABIES IN IT and I couldn't leave them alone. There was no relief. I eventually became completely exhausted and began falling into a very deep sleep as soon as my head hit the pillow. Half an hour later in a half-asleep state, I'd start screaming and ripping the bed-clothes off the bed. There was a baby suffocating under the blankets. It wasn't breathing and I couldn't find it. I'd jump out, pull the bedclothes off completely, then dive under the bed trying to find the baby. Tony would show me the two babies in their cots, it took him a while to realise I was searching for the third. The third baby.

We had some enormous arguments in the middle of the night. We'd half-wake for baby feeding or comforting and both be irritable and very unreasonable and start slinging nasty comments at each other. By morning, neither of us could remember why.

I clearly remember calling Parentline – the parent help phone line – at 3 a.m. one night demanding that they come and take Tony away immediately. They were very patient with me, asking about the twins and talking about how stressful one, let alone two, small babies can be. We had quite a long chat then they suggested I wait until the morning to get rid of him.

At sleep school I was sent to see the hospital shrink who sorted me out in a 45 minute session. I overcame my fear of babies dying and decided our family was going into shutdown mode. I was going to have to be self-ish and look after myself, the girls and Tony. No visitors, no-one else.

ANOTHER MUM SAYS 'Entering into the daily grind of motherhood is a huge adjustment and fundamentally changes our lives. We are often our harshest critics and expect too much from ourselves, our partners and our babies. We naively expect every day to be extraordinary when the reality is very different. Inevitably the daily routine is lots of ordinary mundane chores, with a few short bursts of 'extraordinary' thrown in to keep us going. We ought to stop being so tough on ourselves; we need to learn to pat ourselves on the back for just getting through a day.'

ANOTHER MUM SAYS 'My partner and I have always been interested in sport and current affairs. We manage to spend some time each day talking about something that exists outside the house. It's been an effort at times but I'm sure it's helped ward off the cabin fever and made me more comfortable on the occasions I do socialise.'

Adapting to your new role

Many women describe motherhood as the best thing they ever did, while at times also finding it frustrating, difficult and impossible to get right. We receive little if any training and there may be few tangible rewards, particularly in the early months. Often mothers identify that their work is not recognised and is taken for granted.

Many women find themselves asking 'Who am I?' Things that were such a large part of our lives before having children, like our job, friends, looks, clothes, social life, priorities and choices, generally change completely. Even when things don't seem to change, we feel different because now we have children.

ANOTHER MUM SAYS 'In the first month I remember this overwhelming feeling of grief. I broke down when I was having a massage. I burst into tears and spent over an hour talking to the masseuse about my fears bringing two children into the world, missing my husband (although we were probably together more than ever, we were both dealing with our own shock at the change to our comfortable, free lives), the IVF curse (I should be grateful, grateful, grateful), and the whole bonding thing which wasn't instantaneous as I had imagined. Things do get better and although I half-expected this was just another thing people say, it really is true.'

ANOTHER MUM SAYS 'I try to help prepare my women friends who are contemplating having babies by being brutally frank. I tell them that for 90 per cent of the time they will be the workhorse and the person who does all the hard yards. Forget feminism, especially all those ideologies of equality that we've grown up with. The mothers are the ones who spend all day in the laundry, the bathroom and the kitchen and carry all the responsibility for the babies. We're the ones who lose our work friends, careers and our sense of self.'

Until 30 years ago most women spent most of their time child rearing and homemaking. Modern mothers of twins have the adjustment of gaining two babies to care for, and often, at the same time, losing their professional identity. As a result, new mothers can feel a general lack of confidence. The tiredness and adjustments related to feeding and settling the babies can contribute to many new mothers feeling inadequate. It takes most of us some time and thought to adjust to our new roles.

ANOTHER MUM SAYS 'I've never been happier. Of course there are difficult times, but even after a really hard day I can only remember how lucky I am. I feel truly blessed and while it can be frustrating at times and very hard work, I can't imagine choosing a different life.'

Below are three questions which may help you to think about defining yourself as a mother.

1. What were your expectations of being a mother?

2. What is your actual experience of being a mother?

3. What influences your experience of being a mother?
   e.g. having a multiple birth, your economic circumstances,
   health issues, your own childhood.

It is important for all of us to continue to have a sense of self once we become mothers. One way to develop a stronger sense of self is to have some 'me' time. Those first 12 months in the life of twins is so busy that sometimes organising time-out just feels like something else on the list of things to do.

SOME WAYS TO SPEND TIME ON YOURSELF

- Remember there is no such thing as the perfect mother. Relinquish control and perfection. It is OK to allow someone else to put your babies to bed or to be in charge – it doesn't always have to be you and it doesn't have to be done the way you do it.

- Organise with your partner for each of you to have a regular activity outside the house and away from the family.

- Organise a baby-sitter, occasional care or childcare. Use the time off to do something not related to the household or the babies.

- If your babies usually sleep two hours, try giving the first hour to yourself to do what you choose. Do the household chores in the second hour. If they wake up early, you will still have had time for yourself.

- Plan to do regularly the things you enjoy doing with your babies; shopping, visiting friends, baby sessions at the movies, baby-friendly coffee shops.

ANOTHER MUM SAYS   'Three hours of paid help once a week means I'm regularly temporarily off the treadmill. It's no longer a continuing cycle 24 hours a day, seven days a week. Those three hours away change my outlook towards the children, my partner and even the housework.'

ANOTHER MUM SAYS   'Around 12 months I hit that point where I wanted my old life back. I suddenly missed my lack of freedom and although I wanted my life to change instantly I had neither the means, the support nor the energy to do it. I had a feeling of self-loathing, resentment toward my husband and I didn't feel at all sexual. I'd become the complete antithesis of who I was and I wanted it all back. I realised I needed physical space from the babies to sit down and consider my own situation. With some childcare, gradually, I got back some of the things I lost. Then I learnt that some things I didn't want back – I'd moved on. There's never been a point where I wished I never had them or wish they'd come separately. I focus on the positive and believe that denying a certain amount of the negatives is healthy. I consciously practise keeping perspective and positivism. I know I am much stronger and more capable if I'm not focusing on negative feelings. This has kept me from feeling powerless and depressed at times. However, when I am able to crumble under the hugeness of the situation I talk, I cry, I have a hissy-fit, dust myself off, get help if I need it or have a cuppa if it's just letting off steam. I find talking really helps and talking to twin mums is best. Who else knows what you're going through? I never want the boys to feel that just because they were born at the same time that they were any burden. I want them to feel that they are perfect – which they are.'

Guilt, anxiety, depression and anger

Many women expect to feel similar after the birth of their babies to the way they felt before. Others imagine feeling better. You may have expected to feel delighted and content at all times.

Feelings of depression are more common in parents of multiples than parents of singleton babies. Forty per cent of mothers still had a diagnosis of PND at four years.

Looking after babies is a very demanding and life-changing experience for most women. The work is never ending, isolating and undervalued. This can cause many new mothers to feel depressed or anxious. Those in the paid workforce wouldn't respond well to the same conditions.

Are you depressed or just feeling down?
Common 'mood changes' that can occur following childbirth are:

- **Baby blues:** most women experience some emotional upset and tearfulness during the first days and weeks after the birth of their babies. This is usually attributed to hormones and is often called 'post-partum blues'.
- **Mild depression:** a normal response when adjusting to parenthood and an understandable part of being at home with two babies, particularly when you don't have much support. There are usually emotional peaks and troughs as babies and parents experience sleep problems, relationship issues, financial pressures, inequitable workload and whatever else life throws at us during this time.
- **Postnatal depression (PND):** some health experts find that most women experience some form of depression after the birth of either of their children. Usually PND is diagnosed in moderate to severe cases of depression. Australian statistics vary with from one in five to one in eight women having postnatal depression.
- **Post-partum psychosis:** affects one in 500 women, usually within two weeks of giving birth. It requires urgent medical attention and usually a hospital stay. There is an excellent recovery rate.

ANOTHER MUM SAYS 'I kept getting signals that I wasn't allowed to feel sorry for myself. My doctor thought I needed drugs, but I didn't agree. I felt that I would be making the symptoms go away rather than going through the process of fixing the problem. I just needed someone to talk with, listen and understand. Friends would ring to check I was OK but that made me feel obliged to cheer up, be grateful, be happy.'

When you are feeling depressed you may be experiencing:
- mood changes
- sleep disturbance unrelated to your babies' patterns – bad dreams, insomnia, sleep walking, over-sleeping, sudden waking
- loss of appetite or increased weight gain
- chronic exhaustion or hyperactivity
- crying without knowing why
- feeling unable to cope
- irritability
- sensitivity to noise
- negative, obsessive or morbid thoughts
- feeling that life has no meaning
- anxiety – hot and cold flushes, heart palpitations, dizziness, hyperventilation
- loss of concentration
- loss of memory
- no interest in sex
- loss of self-confidence and self-esteem
- feelings of guilt and inadequacy
- fear of being alone
- fear of social contact

As parents of twins, you may experience many of these symptoms at different times. Does this mean you are feeling depressed? The severity of any of these symptoms along with their impact on your ability to cope day to day are determining factors in diagnosing PND. It's a good idea to discuss your emotions with your maternal child health nurse and ask for a referral to a psychologist. They are professionals in behaviour, feelings and attitude changes.

HELPING THE BABY BLUES
- Have a good cry, then focus on what you have to do now.
- Prepare friends to listen, not to argue or judge. Ask them to remind you of all the things you are doing. Talking about your feelings in an undirected way, going over the same things, can be very unhealthy.
- Don't have visitors unless you want them.
- Understand that feeling overwhelmed and teary is a normal response. Be kind to yourself, ask someone to give you baby-sitting time, a massage, or take you out for lunch.

WHAT CAN HELP MILD DEPRESSION?

- Talking with other parents of twins
- Writing a list of the ways you'd like to look after yourself
- Seeking further information and advice on specific issues like sleeping and feeding (see Resources, pages 340–47)
- Counselling
- Organising some childcare to ensure a proper break from the babies
- Returning to work part-time or full-time

ANOTHER MUM SAYS   'My GP is also a psychologist and three hour-long counselling sessions with her have really helped me deal with my anger and disappointment over the birth and bonding difficulties. I saw her as soon as I recognised that I was feeling uncomfortable with my feelings. Seeking help early probably helped me avoid a descent into depression.'

ANOTHER MUM SAYS   'After I got over the wonderful hormonal high you experience after childbirth and the flowers had died and the visitors had left and it was just me and two babies, I did find motherhood a bit of a shock. I had been a professional woman running my own business for six years and operating at a high level of competency and confidence in a competitive male-dominated profession. Suddenly my world was totally female and totally at the mercy of two tiny dependent beings who I could not control. For an A-type personality this was a huge adjustment. I was financially dependent and operating in a physical realm rather than a cerebral one and I had to be satisfied with achieving small accomplishments like getting to the supermarket or to the baby movie sessions. It took a fair bit of talking with other women and self-analysis to adjust to the maternal world and it's different, more subtle joys.'

Postnatal depression

Australian statistics show that between one in five and one in eight mothers experience postnatal depression. A recent British study showed that the rate of depression among mothers of twins (up to five years old) was 1.5 times higher than mothers of single babies.

Postnatal depression is a reaction to events that objectively seem more severe than the situation warrants. Some women are reluctant to name their experience 'postnatal depression', partly because they don't agree with the 'label' but also because it is hard to admit things aren't rosy. Many depressed mothers tell everyone they are fine. They fear that the label 'postnatal depression' has negative connotations and implies a weakness. It happens to many of us and there is little research as to the actual cause – except that it's a response to this overwhelmingly new situation.

ANOTHER MUM SAYS 'My doctor labelled me as postnatally depressed and wanted to write me out a script straightaway. This quick diagnosis made me feel very uncomfortable. I didn't want to be seen as not coping and I also thought he was jumping to conclusions. I was very tired and emotional but fundamentally happy, not depressed.'

ANOTHER MUM SAYS 'When I tell people how big an adjustment parenthood was for me and how shocked I was by my angry feelings and my ambivalence towards my babies, they ask me if I was post-natally depressed. It's taken me a while but now I'm able to say 'yes' and not feel ashamed. Of course I was depressed, it was an awful situation and I was under great stress, as well as grieving for my old life. I believe depression is a completely normal reaction in response to becoming a new mother of either one or two babies.'

SYMPTOMS OF POSTNATAL DEPRESSION

- Inner withdrawal where everybody else is 'out there' – this can include withdrawing from your babies
- Feeling numb or like a robot
- Excessive crying
- Anxiety, panic attacks or heart palpitations
- Feeling overwhelmed by anxiety
- No energy to care for babies or yourself
- Physical symptoms that do not respond to treatment, such as headaches, digestive disorders and chronic pain
- Difficulty concentrating, remembering or making decisions
- Feeling hopeless, worthless or constantly pessimistic
- Thoughts of death or suicide
- Suicide attempts

The defining characteristic of feeling depressed is the lack of happy or positive feelings. If you experience several of the symptoms for longer than a couple of weeks or, if the symptoms interfere with your daily routine, it's time to seek help.

Doctors classify postnatal depression as an 'illness' from which we need to 'recover' with the assistance of antidepressants. While medication may ease some of the symptoms and help increase energy to fight the depression, it can be more beneficial when used in conjunction with counselling and professional support. Psychologists identify what we need to learn to do to cope with this incredibly difficult and overwhelming situation.

Postnatal depression can put an enormous strain on any partnership, even when the partners are patient, loving and supportive. It isn't unusual for a couple battling PND to think that their relationship is beyond repair. The good news is that most relationships return to normal once the depression lifts.

Where to get help

Exercise is the single biggest factor in alleviating feelings of depression. Yoga and long walks are excellent. Support and patience from family and friends is crucial in recovery. Talking about your feelings, particularly with other women in support groups or to a psychologist, can be incredibly helpful. Antidepressants and other medications might be recommended to help bring about a change in mood.

> **YOU CAN GET HELP FOR PND FROM**
> a psychologist
> a PND support group
> your GP

ANOTHER MUM SAYS   'I had no postnatal depression with my first child. With the twins it crept up on me. I think it was because things weren't going as well as they had first time round. I was such a routine person, and the twins had different rules to mine! I thought because it was so hard that I was doing something wrong. When they were about nine months old I started crying and was not able to deal with anything. I could function and when people visited I pretended I was fine. I felt resentful that my best friend couldn't look at me and know. But she didn't. My husband knew something was wrong. He didn't know when he came home from work whether I'd be crying and he'd have to deal with me all night. I'm forever grateful that he decided to call my GP and get help. It was so different from anything I'd ever dealt with emotionally. After seeing my GP, who referred me to a specialist, I was prescribed an antidepressant. I felt better after talking to the specialist and then the medication worked in a couple of days. I don't mind taking antidepressants, but other people's judgements are irritating when they have no idea what they are talking about. I think it was my hormones altering brain chemicals and the situation compounded these feelings.'

Anger management

Some parents are surprised at how angry they feel. They usually also feel guilty for being and sounding angry with their babies. Realising it's the situation rather than the babies deliberately trying to frustrate you, helps to get things in perspective. Feelings of anger can mask depression. Seek help if you are concerned about your feelings.

IN MOMENTS OF ANGER:
- Stop what you're doing.
- Put the babies down somewhere safe – **never shake your babies**.
- Take a deep breath.
- Think about why you're angry. Maybe it's because they're crying or because you're frustrated about not being able to stop it.
- Write down your thoughts. Look for words and statements like:
  - should or shouldn't have, must have, got to, need to
  - awful, terrible
  - I can't stand it, can't bear it
  - they're so awful, they're little brats
- Identify how you're feeling – is it angry, guilty, anxious, depressed?
- Do something to help clear your head so you can think what to do. Go outside for five minutes by yourself or take a shower. Exercise is fantastic, take a brisk walk around the block, bike ride to the shops or do 50 star-jumps.

- Draw a picture of yourself being angry and make it look ridiculous.
- Recall the last time you were angry and how useless it was, how it didn't change anything for the better.
- Know the anger will pass.
- When you calm down a bit, you will be better able to work out what to do next – cuddle your babies, sing them a song, make dinner.
- Take another deep breath if they start crying again.

THE BEST THINGS ABOUT HAVING TWINS

- It's a great conversation starter – in fact you don't need any other topics.
- You have an instant family.
- You'll be the centre of attention wherever you go.
- You'll have a special bond with other parents of twins – a shared roller-coaster experience.
- There are no arguments about who holds the baby – you've got one each.
- It's so incredibly special when your twins laugh together for the first time.
- Watching them interact provides non-stop entertainment – playing peek-a-boo together and discovering each others belly buttons!
- You never finish meals or do anything sitting down so you lose weight – supposedly.
- You give and receive twice the love, the kisses and the cuddles.
- Both your babies have an instant playmate so there's less chance of them clinging to you.
- By the time they turn three they'll be keeping each other company while you're busy with the new baby.

TIPS FOR SURVIVING BEING A MOTHER

- Acknowledge it's all right to feel angry sometimes.
- Recognise that you are in a stressful situation.
- Know you will feel well and happy again.
- Stop covering up your feelings and talk honestly to family, friends and professionals.
- Accept that mothers give out a lot of energy to their babies, their partner and managing the household and little, if any, to themselves.
- Plan some realistic goals for short-term objectives and feel good when you've achieved them.
- Plan to do at least one small thing for yourself every day.
- Speak up when you are doing more than you can manage.
- Accept that there will sometimes be bad days and bad moments.
- Have days where you all lie around in your PJs and watch videos.
- If you've done something you regret and are experiencing guilt, that is positive and healthy for a short time. Then forgive yourself for your mistakes.

TIPS FOR PARTNERS

- If you suspect your partner is suffering from PND, seek help.
- Listen to her without judgement.
- Tell her regularly you love her, don't assume she knows it. Many women feel unlovable and need to know their partners aren't going to leave them.
- Set limits on visitors by saying 'no' when she's not up to company.
- Accept all genuine offers of help by friends or family.
- Do as many of the household tasks as you can.
- Be physically affectionate without asking for sex.
- Don't usurp her role – she may need precise help and support but should be encouraged to continue in mothering her babies.
- Provide positive feedback for any achievements.
- Look after yourself too – take time for something you enjoy.
- Find someone to talk to.

Dynamics and dynamite

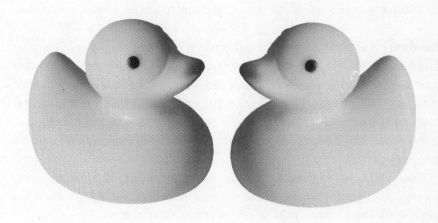

RELATIONSHIPS

RELATIONSHIPS: OUR STORIES

Relationships with your partner, members of your family and friends can change when you become a parent and sometimes more so when you add more than one child to the family. Having twins is demanding and team work is far more productive than warfare, but when you're exhausted it's harder to make an effort with people. And they are adjusting to the changes in your life as well. Suddenly, conversations may revolve around your children, shopping, cooking and housework. The amount of time you spend with particular people may also change. Time spent with some friends or relatives may increase, while you may spend less time with others.

Katrina: I had no idea that having children would impact on our marriage. I was completely surprised that becoming parents just gave us reasons to fight. After seven strong years together the first 12 months of the babies' lives was the most challenging time in our relationship. The babies were now the priority, not each other. It was no longer about me!

Louise: I was feeling mentally responsible for absolutely everything; the finances and bill paying, the shopping, doctor's appointments, childcare planning, drop-offs and pick-ups, birthdays and our social arrangements. And we both had paid jobs. I asked my partner to take on the mental responsibility for cooking and house cleaning. If he wanted me do anything other than clean up after myself, he had to ask me. It really took the pressure off.

Every time we started to bicker during that first 12 months, we'd remind each other that we're on the same team. Sometimes the situation pushed us into behaving like enemies rather than partners.

ANOTHER DAD SAYS   'When the babies were born, my dreams were extinguished. Even though they were only fantasies, it was possible for me to believe I had choices. Suddenly my entire future was mapped out. It took almost two years for me to stop resenting my lack of freedom and to fully appreciate the intense satisfaction my family brings.'

Your partner

When your babies arrive there will be more to do and less time to do it in. Your partner may be better at expecting and taking time-out. Adding up who has done more, is more tired, or has a harder role achieves nothing and causes resentment. It may be better to think about what you would like and to work out together how this can be managed. This may require some frank discussion about expectations and needs of each partner. It may be wise to do this before the babies are born and before you both get too exhausted to think straight.

ANOTHER MUM SAYS 'I always feel like I should be doing more rather than less. How can I escape to a movie when there is washing to be folded, lunches to be packed and a bank of sewing. He's not going to do it. I hate the 'help' word. By looking after his children for an hour he thinks he's 'helping' me and giving me a break. It's his job too. The worst thing is I feel obliged to thank him for it. I don't get thanked for all the hours I give.'

ANOTHER MUM SAYS 'I feel I can't complain because he's so good with the babies ...'

ANOTHER MUM SAYS 'For a long time I was envious of my partner. He still got to go off to stimulating work everyday and enjoy expensive lunches and socialise with interesting people. His life didn't seem much different, except for his baby bit at the beginning or the end of the day – which had actually enhanced his life. Meanwhile I just felt more locked into the routine, and locked out of my 'old' life.'

ANOTHER DAD SAYS 'I had two children born two years apart in my first marriage so I imagined twins would be much the same. Society understands to some extent the pressures on the mother of twins, but as the father I felt completely unsupported. I'm financially responsible for the family, work more than 40 hours a week, then come home to a second job. It's utterly relentless. I take time-out watching TV at night but this just adds to my tiredness the next day.'

ANOTHER MUM SAYS 'I know I've been my own worst enemy, reinforcing the status quo. I want a break yet I want to be the one with the children. There's a struggle between my innate female nurturing side and my modern self-actualising persona. Often I resent him when I feel I need a break but at the same time I can't let go.'

Difficult situations are exaggerated with twins. If you'd like to change the way things are working in your home, the responsibility for changing belongs to both of you. Most parents put their children before themselves and defer their own needs. It may take time to get any sense of work-family-self balance. When you're breastfeeding, there is usually a two-hour window available. Learn to grab it and do things that only take two hours but can change your mood; a book club, a movie, tennis, swimming or spending time alone.

- Talk with each other about what each of you and your children need.
- Write a list of needs and wants and work out when to give each parent time off.
- Weigh up whether you can afford to spend some money on domestic help.
- Your partner may be good at doing what they're told – but may need instructions. Try to ask nicely rather than snarl or yell.
  Then try to let your partner be a parent without your interference.

ANOTHER MUM SAYS 'I was feeling frustrated that he just didn't understand the enormous effort involved in getting through every day. I decided on a plan to get the message across. He was very keen to arrive on time at a Grand Final barbecue. Ten minutes before we were due there, I put my shoes and coat on, announced that I was ready and went out and sat in the passenger seat of the car. He finally got everyone and everything into the car. We were 45 minutes late. Since then he has always helped me get the kids ready.'

ANOTHER MUM SAYS 'Our husbands all have Friday night drinks so we do too. I pack up the four kids and take them out with the girls for drinks every Friday. We go to an indoor play-land from 4 to 6 p.m. and we can take our own drinks. There's always someone to hold a baby. We get the kids a bowl of chips for dinner and everybody's happy.'

In a 1992 study of nearly 100 couples, 97 per cent reported more conflict after the arrival of a baby. Despite the increase in conflict, couples are more committed to each other once they become parents. The arrival of the first child or children can give the parents a real sense of being a family, with their bond strengthened by their joint creation. Initially these feelings can be very strong. Sometimes when domestic life takes over it can be difficult to keep the big picture in mind.

Many couples start out planning to co-parent and share the workload, yet something often happens to those good intentions. Once children arrive, Australian couples tend to conform closely to the gender stereotype. The pattern of the relationship changes and generally it's the mother's role that changes most. Often the mother does the housework, the cooking, the shopping, tidying up, pays the bills, coordinates and implements social activities and has the huge responsibility of caring for the children.

The mother can also carry the responsibility for all the planning, remembering and organising: the 'mental work of parenting', as well as most of the physical parenting work. The partner's role often concentrates on being the financial provider. The most common concern raised by fathers of twins is their constant feeling of guilt. They feel guilty about not managing well at work and feel guilty about not pulling their weight at home.

Some couples adapt smoothly to parenthood. For others, tiredness and stress can cause them to become distant and withdrawn. Becoming parents means there is less time for each other. While many people adapt easily to these changes, others feel left out or unloved. Happiness in your relationship is an important part of your personal happiness. The transition into parenthood is a major turning point for most relationships and even more so for parents of twins. Partners who don't actively participate are more likely to feel left out and to seek other forms of satisfaction either at work or in relationships outside the home.

Statistics show that the incidence of relationship breakdown is greater in parents of multiples not only following the birth of twins but at the time of diagnosis and before the birth. Some parents can feel overwhelmed by the responsibilities.

Time and emotional energy is channelled away from the couple's relationship and put into parenting. Affection previously shared with each other is now being poured onto the children. Partners can feel resentful of the babies and frightened that the demands placed on them have greatly increased as they deal with babies, an emotional partner and their work life. Parental teamwork can make a big difference. Unlike some families with one child, with twins, the partner is usually involved right from the beginning. Most partners learn to enjoy their participation in day-to-day care which also means the mother copes better, siblings are less likely to feel left out and the family functions better.

It's very difficult to negotiate new household arrangements and fair parenting when you're also tired and cranky. Try not to do it when you're angry or during an argument. Make a time to discuss it the following day when you've calmed down and thought about what you'd like to say.

ANOTHER MUM SAYS   'Our relationship has deepened so much since the birth of the boys. I have such a trust and love for him that is so much deeper than I could have ever imagined. Having twins has really tested us but we know we'll look back on this time and say what a great job we did. There have been times when we've resented each other because each of our roles are so invisible and thankless and just expected. While as a mother my job never ends, equally his role as the main breadwinner is also endless because the money goes out as quickly as it comes in. It's hard to appreciate yourself, let alone the other person. There are few immediate rewards for the sacrifices parents make. It's a big adjustment to go from buying yourself cases of wine to cask plonk, or from having a massage twice a month or going to the movies when you fancy. Everything has to be negotiated and planned much more than before kids. The lack of spontaneity is unsexy. We'd talk about how we felt and sometimes just saying the words is enough ... sometimes I resent this. We'd understand each other because we usually both felt the same way. We have always had a will to make things right and a cup of tea together and a cuddle goes a long way. It helps us to put things in perspective. We have two perfect healthy boys and we don't live in a war-torn, ravaged place. Things could always be worse. You've got to be so strong and try to maintain a sense of humour. Seventeen months in and we're still just getting used to being parents. We're operating more smoothly as a family now. Our roles are fairly defined and we know what each other is expected to do.'

Strengthening your relationship

These are some steps which may help you strengthen your relationship with your partner:

- Share your experiences – talk about the joys and achievements, as well as your doubts and frustration. Let each other know how you feel.
- Take control of your relationship – be clear about how you want your relationship to be and how you would like your new family to be. Talk about family traditions and values that are important to you.
- Give yourself time – spend time alone together as a couple, regularly and without your children. This will give you a chance to get close and recharge your batteries. How often you spend time without your babies will depend on your circumstances. You could aim for an evening a month, and a weekend away once or twice a year once the babies are old enough. If family support isn't available, try a trusted friend with children around the same age with whom you can take turns.
- Accept practical support from others – it protects you from divorce.

(ANOTHER MUM SAYS) 'We have a date at 7.30 p.m. every Saturday night. The kids are in bed, the TV's off. We have a glass of wine and a chat. It's amazing how half an hour really dissolves the friction. At 8.00 p.m, I'm off to bed and the TV is back on.'

If you find that you have continuing difficulties and disappointments in your relationship after becoming parents, consider seeking help through counselling. It often helps talking to someone who understands some of the changes you have been going through, who can help you and your partner communicate more clearly. Again, other parents of twins can be a great source of understanding and advice.

Communication

Typical traits in families that function well include positive communication, respect, spending time together and working as a team.

Many of us are great communicators and listeners in our professional lives. Using these communication skills in your personal life helps your relationship evolve and you cope better with the pressures of your new lifestyle. Just as you would in your workplace when you have an issue to raise, you can make an appointment with your partner and indicate the subject you'd like to talk about. This sounds very business-like but it does give you both a chance to think about some of the issues and discuss them at a time that is mutually convenient, rather than while eating dinner or as soon as your partner walks in the door. For example, 'I want us to talk tonight. Shall we do that at about 8.30 when the children are in bed?' It's a nicer way to start a discussion than screaming.

Practise using 'I' statements rather than making accusations. Starting a discussion with an 'I' statement helps the other person see your point of view. It also means you're less likely to be critical and call each other names. 'I feel hurt when you sit there while there's washing to be folded.' ' I don't think that you're supporting my decision to breastfeed' rather than a 'you' statement such as 'You don't do anything around here' or 'You make me do it all'. This will only work if you are functioning well as a couple. If you are in conflict it will probably just start another argument. First you need to focus on getting the relationship right.

> ANOTHER MUM SAYS 'I'm terrible at always looking for the
> meaning in what he says. He might say, 'This place is a mess' and
> I immediately jump into justifying why I haven't had a chance to
> clean it up yet and get cross with him, saying, 'I'm doing my best'
> when all he said was 'It's a mess' and I could have just agreed.
> I would add the layers of meaning which weren't really there.'

Try to acknowledge the other person's feelings. We feel the way we feel. No one can tell us how we should feel. We need to be able to express negative as well as positive emotions. If you're angry and upset, the last thing that helps is someone telling you there's no need to be. What usually helps most is that someone has listened to us and acknowledges our feelings. 'I can see that you're upset because you don't think I'm doing enough.' You might not agree with the other person, but it may help to understand what it is that they are feeling. 'I don't want to upset you.'

If you want to talk about your relationships with someone objective, you could try your GP, local community health centre, parenting helpline or psychologist. Contact details for organisations offering relationship guidance are given in Resources, pages 340–47.

Unsettled partners

Although the mother usually has more obvious physical and emotional changes to adjust to with the arrival of twins, partners can suffer from depression too as a result of sleep deprivation and pressures of work and family life. This is more common in families with twins.

> (ANOTHER MUM SAYS) 'I'm watching my husband play with our gorgeous girls who are now over two and a half years old. It is almost impossible to associate this relaxed and happy man with the person who nearly 'broke down' when they were infants. My husband did not cope well with the pressures associated with caring for two newborns. If there is an equivalent, he believes that he suffered a male version of postnatal depression. He felt instantly overwhelmed from the moment they were born. We went from a tight unit of three to a big noisy family of five; suddenly it was difficult to move freely … without taking half the house with us. While he was an excellent father, as for many men the day-to-day baby chores were frustrating and a hassle. This became the crux of many future issues; I had so diligently coped with our first baby, why couldn't I cope as well with another two? He really seemed to resent my needing his constant assistance and would often tease me that I wasn't coping. I resented always having to ask for his help.
>
> To add to my husband's growing stress, our twin babies were very unsettled, especially at night. Once they woke, they could cry for hours. We suffered terrible sleep deprivation and our marriage came under pressure. My husband found the twins' persistent crying a constant source of aggravation. There were times when he would return home from work and just stand on the doorstep listening to the wailing coming from inside. He told me that on many occasions his instinct was to run. Of course the moment he entered the house, I would pounce on him and hand him a baby so that I could finish getting dinner ready. I was aware that he wasn't coping and that he had a growing resentment for these demanding little creatures who had turned our house upside down. I was desperate for him to dote on the twins with the same affection he had always showered on our first daughter. My emotions were torn. I felt guilty asking for his help if this was going to make him resent the twins more. I felt angry that this help didn't naturally come. I felt betrayed that he was expecting me to be the 'strong one' … I had never really been given any choice.

As the months passed, my husband began to make me feel responsible for the twin's unsettled behaviour, or at least responsible for a solution. As I was breastfeeding them, his response to every whimper was 'put them on the boob, they must be hungry.' I'd just fed them. 'Well, put them on the boob anyway, that will shut them up.' The twins seemed to bring out the worst in him and this filled me with despair. Equally, he seemed to bring out the worst in them. It was as though they sensed his impatience and general lack of enthusiasm towards them. If I needed to go out on my own, leaving the babies with him, he would panic and immediately place restrictions on me. I felt as though I was the one holding the family together, 24 hours a day.

The worst emotion that this situation brought out was hate. I hated my husband's inability to cope with his babies. We fought a lot about the imbalance of responsibility, especially in regard to night time 'shifts'; certainly I was breastfeeding but the nappy changes and general settling could have been more evenly shared. He argued that he was constantly tired by the demands of the twins and needed to function effectively during the day at work. I argued that I couldn't go all day and all night on my own. Most of the time, he was oblivious to the amount of times I'd be up and down, in and out of bed to our wailing babies. Sometimes I stood my ground and refused to be the one to get up all night. I'd physically shake him awake and demand that he take over. Most of the time this was a pointless exercise; he would go into their room in a stupor and desperately try to settle them, stumbling from cot to cot with no hope of calming them down. He would quickly become more anxious and would upset them more. He really struggled to deal with them because they were two. It was for this reason that he hated to be left alone with them for any length of time; he felt helpless when they both needed him at once. As little babies they were breastfed, so he couldn't settle them with bottles. They refused to take dummies. He felt as though he had no control over the situation, rendering him powerless. I understood this and felt sorry for him. However, his apprehension was preventing him from enjoying his babies; he was focusing on the negative all the time and this was contributing to his depression.

Fortunately, we have always communicated well. Throughout this difficult time we constantly expressed our emotions, even if it led to arguments and tears. He knew that I felt that he had abandoned me. Prior to having our twins, our relationship had never been challenged. I never thought it possible, but I was seeing the limit of his love for me; a love that I had always regarded as unconditional. I was deeply hurt and felt that I would never forgive him for being so selfish. Certainly, our twins were hard work but there was also a lot of pleasure to be gained from them. He let his intolerance and impatience cloud this.

After about eight months, things began to change for the better and tensions began to melt away. Our tiny babies were blossoming into irresistible little girls and my husband's genuine displays of affection emerged. This brought me such pleasure. He was finally really enjoying them and accepting them for who they were. It was as though he'd given up the 'fight' and was at last surrendering to their demands – good and bad.

Our relationship has taken a beating since the birth of our twins. Some 18 months later I could still be reduced to tears when we talked about how he struggled to come to terms with having twins. Through it all we have certainly learnt a lot about each other. Because we have openly 'hashed over' our anger and disappointment, we have moved on in a positive way. This would be my strongest advice to all couples expecting twins; always keep the channels of communication open and try to define your expectations of each other before the babies come along. After your twins are born, try to get time away together as a couple to talk. Sometimes you need to do this just to remind yourself of why you fell in love in the first place.'

Sex

Our relationships are also affected by changes in our desire for sex. Having twins can change your sex life. Your body has probably changed. Your tummy may still be soft and wobbly, your breasts could be tender and you may have a vaginal discharge for many weeks. If you had an episiotomy or caesarean you could also be in some physical pain.

Theoretically, sex is more of an option around six weeks after the birth. In practice, it's unlikely many parents of twins will get around to it regularly for some time yet. You may be physically and emotionally exhausted just caring for your babies. If you've cuddled them all day and at night, it's not surprising you don't feel like cuddling anyone else.

Women vary greatly in their needs or desire for sex during pregnancy and after the birth. Any level of depression can also reduce your sex drive. Women often say that they need to feel good about themselves and their partner, in order to want to have sex. If you're tired and stressed, sex may just feel like another thing you have to do.

> (ANOTHER MUM SAYS)   'I wanted to have sex and I didn't want to have sex. It took months for my episiotomy scar to heal and I had leaky breasts and jelly belly. I felt like my vagina had been trauma- tised and needed to be left alone for a tad. The idea of a penis inside me was far too much. I also felt my vagina was much bigger than it used to be and felt I'd aged so quickly. My lack of sexual urge was very much related to my own body image and it's been hard for me to accept my permanent physical changes. My partner was very kind and didn't place any demands on me and we kept being really affectionate. Gradually I became less sensitive to my new body but I think our sex life will never be what it was. I'm not sure. It's a work in progress. I'm still finding my place as a mother, a sexual being and an owner of a jelly belly. I contemplated plastic surgery but feel that it's a 'sacred site' – my badge of motherhood. I'll try to resist the urge.'

It may help to talk about sex with your partner so that you both know what the other is thinking and feeling. We often feel relieved if we know it's not personal, and that many women rarely feel like sex in the early years of motherhood.

If sex isn't a high priority for you at present, it is still vital for your relationship that you remain intimate. Tell your partner you love them. Turn off the TV and do something special together. Sex can wait until you're ready.

Sorting out contraception is an important part of returning to a sex life. Talk to your GP about contraception options. Breastfeeding women also usually experience a dry vagina so keep the water-based lubricant handy just in case you're suddenly in the mood. Sex doesn't have to be a night-time-in-bed-activity. If you're more energetic in the day, then maybe there's a window of opportunity for some 'parent' time.

(ANOTHER MUM SAYS) 'We didn't have sex until the girls were over 12 months old and after I stopped breastfeeding. I was terrified of the prospect of getting pregnant. The only 100 per cent effective contraception is abstinence. It was really nice to get back into it and a relief not to feel guilty about our celibacy anymore.'

Colliding careers

Mothers work outside the home more than ever before, but continue to be the main carers and are responsible for most of the household tasks. A 1999 Australian study examining the distribution of housework showed that mothers, whether in paid work or not, contributed 70–80 per cent of the time spent on housework and childcare. The study also showed that those working full-time did the same amount of the household jobs as mothers not in paid work.

If they go back to work, women who do that second shift when they get home feel constantly 'at work'. Juggling these roles can be stressful and exhausting. Many mothers feel a lack of control when something disturbs the routine, like a sick child or a house-guest. Even when something fabulous happens, it alters the balance and life can suddenly become chaos.

(ANOTHER MUM SAYS) 'Now that I've returned to work, our redefined roles are a constant source of argument. He still seems to think that the fairy godmother is going to look after all the washing and cooking.'

(ANOTHER MUM SAYS) 'We both have busy jobs yet when the babies are sick the assumption is that I'll be the one who stays home to look after them.'

(ANOTHER MUM SAYS) 'We decided if we never bought takeaways we could afford a cleaner for two hours a week. It's not much but I think it saved our marriage.'

(ANOTHER MUM SAYS) 'It might not be equal, but by partner does the dishes every night which means a clean kitchen every day.'

Same-sex couples

Lesbian mothers of twins may experience additional challenges to the pregnancy and parenting roller coaster. These may include having to constantly 'come out' to individuals and health professionals and hospital staff with mixed reactions and attitudes. Finding open and suitable professionals and informal groups may also be more complex but important in supporting the new family.

Older children

You may love your children, but it is still possible to feel frustrated and angry with them during the difficult times. As you adapt to parenthood and the challenges of managing two babies, it is common to have ambivalent feelings about older children as well as the babies.

> ANOTHER MUM SAYS   'I have felt resentful of people wanting me to put on a brave face when I've been desperately tired, fearful, and guilty about the lack of time I've had for my daughter. However, it must be said that I perhaps expected people to fully comprehend the situation. This is an unfair expectation. I have been blessed with help and love from close family and friends. At eight months the picture is rosier! I feel totally connected and in love with my boys. The babies are thriving and my daughter is a very happy girl.'

Research into the effect of twins on their siblings shows that there can be problems for siblings in the first few years after the twins arrive. Those born before twins have to make a greater adjustment to the birth of two babies rather than one, and often find it more difficult to cope with the greater reduction in available time from parents while dealing with the attention twins attract. Recent research suggests that when there was more than one child in the family the older children were better able to deal with the situation. If there was another sibling close in age, they often formed another pair. A single older child tended to look outside the family for companionship or attempted to form an alliance with one of the twins to split the pair apart.

Your older children may have mixed feelings about the new arrivals. They might feel they should love the babies but feel confused because they also feel angry. You might like to recognise and discuss their feelings with them.

- If possible, give your other children attention when they ask for it.
- Many parents enjoy having some regular time with older children without their babies – a bedtime story or a trip to the park. Telling them in advance means they can plan their special time.
- Show them photos of themselves as babies.
- If they want to, let them help where possible. Even if it takes longer, their involvement usually pays off.

ANOTHER MUM SAYS 'Five minutes with my older son when he asks for it is worth more than half an hour if he's told to wait till I'm ready.'

ANOTHER MUM SAYS 'Once we took the babies home, we knew our five-year-old daughter would be able to hold them, help with the bottle-feeding (only one baby was being breastfed) and assist with bathing. My partner and I tried so hard to make her a part of this new life but she still found it a huge adjustment. The babies are now 18 months old and things have improved considerably. She now sees them as 'playable' children, even if it is on their terms. Our daughter is a great help to us now and we constantly tell her how lucky we are to have her and point out that it's not just because we need her assistance. We love and value her for her own unique personality and the joy she has brought to our lives. Some days she is harder work than the twins, particularly when she wants attention when a nappy is being changed, a twin is crying or a fight is breaking out amongst the youngest tribe members. We do most things as a whole family now, although we do try to give her time without the twins. Each night I enjoy 'special time' with her, a half an hour that we spend together uninterrupted. We both love this time and look forward to it as it reinforces to our daughter how important and wanted she is. My partner works from home, and he makes time each day to play with her at whatever she chooses (seeing a grown man play with Barbies is quite a sight).'

ANOTHER MUM SAYS 'Our daughter really needs some time away from the babies. When they both cry she sits in a corner with her hands over her ears wishing it would stop. Sometimes I just pop them in their pram and let them scream outside while she and I have some special time together and I can comfort her. Helpful friends and family also give her some one-on-one time my mother takes her every week for a sleepover and she loves it, being the only special one. It also allows me to spend time openly cuddling the boys, lying on the floor with them singing songs and kissing their gorgeous cheeks over and over. I simply can't do this with her in the room. She wants to join in and it usually ends with me having to move the babies away from flailing limbs and over exuberant cuddles. I love this time alone with my babies. It's very important.'

ANOTHER MUM SAYS   'As our daughter was only three when our twins were born, it was difficult to prepare her for the arrival of her baby sisters. It's not as though we could sit down with her and discuss any potential issues that she might have. Certainly we talked to her about mummy's growing tummy and we tried to explain about how the babies would change life in our house, but her understanding was fairly limited. To some degree we were complacent about the impact the twins arrival would have on her. We were more concerned about our own survival! Boy, were we in for a rude awakening!

Our first daughter had been a 'dream' baby – great sleeper, great feeder, easy nature, truly textbook in every way. She sailed through the terrible twos without a tantrum and when we found we were expecting twins she was starting to become independent. Stupidly I expected two more just like her, and I didn't imagine that she could change.

After the twins were born, our daughter instantly regressed in many ways. She had been completely toilet-trained but began wetting herself several times a day. She deliberately misbehaved to get our attention, adopting baby-like habits and suddenly refusing to be independent. Instinctively we understood why she was reacting this way. Her whole world had been turned upside down. We were constantly sensitive to her needs and pandered to her demands as best we could. We insisted that she get extra time with relatives, such as our parents, to cater to her need for one-on-one attention. It seemed the more we gave, the more she expected of us and the worse her behaviour became. The experts said we were responding to her correctly – be patient, kind, understanding, don't make a fuss and she'll improve. After eight weeks we realised that she was perceiving this as a green flag to continue misbehaving. 'Mummy and daddy don't seem to really mind. It gets me the attention I want. This works.' Finally we got angry and showed her that we could no longer tolerate her naughty ways. Within days she realised how serious we were and went back to using the toilet and trying to cooperate more.

In retrospect I think she coped very well. She had to adjust suddenly to changes in her consistent environment. Sure, we were adjusting too, but at least we had maturity on our side. As parents we could have made more effort to talk to other parents of twins and siblings. This may have saved us some time and heartache. However, we were always conscious of including and responding to our child's needs. You do the best you can at the time and sometimes it's easier to relax and deal with each situation as it arises. Also, in the long run sometimes the only 'cure' is time and space to adjust to the impact twins inevitably have on the family.'

Other family members

Your relationships with other members of your family may be altered when your babies arrive. Often the mother/daughter relationship is strengthened after childbirth as a greater understanding and respect develops. But sometimes the opposite is true. New mothers also report feeling disappointed at the lack of support or encouragement, and in some cases disapproval from their own mothers.

If your own siblings have had children, talk to them about how you are feeling. They often make great confidantes even though you might be feeling incompetent. You shouldn't have to be polite with brothers and sisters. If your siblings don't have children, you could involve them as much as they want to be in your babies' lives – it's a great investment in the future.

If your brothers, sisters and parents are willing, they may make excellent baby-sitters or at least 'playing' guests. It benefits children to have close relationships with other special people, whether they are friends, family or childcare providers.

ANOTHER MUM SAYS   'I was shocked and relieved when my loving and supportive mother told me she always thought she would have had a happy life should she not have been able to have children. Shocked to realise I wasn't the centre of her world. Relieved because neither did I feel my kids were the centre of mine.'

ANOTHER MUM SAYS 'I was looking forward finally to having something in common with my mother, but when I was finding motherhood difficult the only comment I got from her was about how good my babies were and how lucky I was. I wanted her to acknowledge that it was really hard work but she just wouldn't.'

Friends

Your babies are likely to preoccupy you so your relationship with friends can change. Establishing friendships with other mothers with children of similar ages can fill gaps but try to continue an interest with some friends who have nothing to do with your children.

Most councils have local mothers' groups and playgroups. AMBA provides a ready-made network of parents of twins. If you connect with someone, pursue their friendship. They're probably as keen as you are to meet other new parents.

ANOTHER MUM SAYS 'As an older mother, I'm in the unusual situation where my friends are all past screaming babies. Their children are at school and mine are still in a pram.'

ANOTHER MUM SAYS 'I wanted to avoid the 'mumsy' thing but got very lonely and really needed to get out of the house. I joined a playgroup and made more social contacts which was good for me and the girls. I've learned more from other women than from health professionals.'

TIPS FOR SURVIVING RELATIONSHIPS

- Talk to your partner about your feelings – talk about sex even if you're not doing it.
- Try not be accusatory when communicating with your partner – proceed gently to start really talking.
- Do special activities with your older children. Involve them in the care of the babies.
- Look for friendships with people in a similar situation to you, but try not to lose touch with your old friends.
- Accept that relationships will change because of the arrival of your twins.
- Seek professional help about the state of your relationship if you are not coping.

TIPS FOR PARTNERS

- Keep the lines of communication open at all times, no matter how exhausted or cross you are. Try pretending you're not.
- Let your partner know how you are feeling about the changes in your lives.
- Make special time for your older children.
- Talk to other parents of twins about what they went through.
- Talk to a counsellor if you need to.

The blurry period

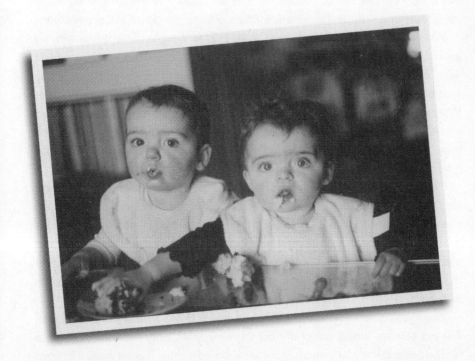

SLEEP

SLEEP: OUR STORIES

Everyone needs sleep, some of us more than others. Plenty of sleep for all can go a long way to making a family happy. For busy parents of twins, there's nothing quite like putting your babies into bed for the night and knowing it's until morning.

Some families find no routine necessary and are quite happy with a situation others would find unbearable. Of course, there are no rules, but if you are, or are about to become, a parent of twins and would like to prepare for getting as much rest as you can, then the guidelines in this chapter may help. Some routines and set approaches to sleep may help your children to establish good sleeping patterns and can help to avoid sleep problems in the future.

Katrina: In hospital I thought my girls were good sleepers. That was because they weren't in my room. They may have been crying and upset but I didn't know about it. They would fall asleep at the end of an hour-long feed and I'd put them back in their cribs in the Special Care Nursery.

When I got our babies home it wasn't as simple. They only stayed awake long enough to be changed and fed, but they slept in an unsettled way. We were nervous that they would wake each other, so if one baby made a peep we'd be in to settle her before she upset her sister. Whenever one was restless we'd go in and soothe her. I tried putting something I'd worn in the cot so the girls could smell me, but they still took turns crying and we ran in popping dummies back in, singing lullabies, patting them and reassuring them.

From the start we began teaching our babies the difference between day and night. When they woke at night we kept it dark and quiet, during the day we played. We'd often grab the upset baby out of her cot at night and pop her into a rocker next to our bed so we could soothe her. We couldn't relax if we had a baby in bed with us. They went straight to sleep in their rockers. I slept whenever I could and usually managed eight hours a day in snatches, rarely more than an hour and a half at a time.

The babies woke properly at least every three hours for their feed. They'd scream while we changed their nappies and set them up for a feed. It was quite a shock after six weeks when they stayed awake longer and needed settling to get to sleep. We were tired and needed them to sleep so that we could. We both got angry very quickly when they wouldn't settle and didn't understand why they seemed to cry for no reason. I didn't know how to make them happy when cuddling and walking around with them didn't work. I did offer the breast occasionally as a settling technique. Sometimes it worked, usually it didn't.

Sometimes I felt so frustrated I swore at my babies. I was unable to keep them happy and had no idea what they wanted. People kept telling me that a baby never died from crying, but I found the crying unbearable.

We were tired and cranky parents, and shouted at each other regularly. We argued about why the babies were crying and about how we should deal with it – meanwhile they screamed in the background. Why would you ever choose to do this to yourself and to your relationship? I kept apologising to Brad because I was the one that had wanted a baby. I'd felt I'd made the biggest mistake of my life.

Through a combination of reading books on sleep and advice from my maternal health nurse, I learnt some settling techniques that calmed my babies and helped me to teach them to sleep. Rather than picking them up and leaving their bedroom or rocking them to sleep in our arms, we put them into their cots awake and settled them in their cots. The techniques we used included patting their bottoms and stroking their foreheads in a soothing way. Their cries and sobs would subside fairly quickly and when they were quiet, we'd leave the room. We left the room before they fell asleep. If they were really distressed, we cuddled them while standing by the cot, giving the firm message that they weren't going to be picked up. If they started up again, we repeated the process. I say 'they' but it was usually one or the other, rarely both. They were usually both asleep within half an hour. As they got used to it, we'd just pop them in their cots, shut their door and they'd happily go to sleep.

During the day they had no set pattern until they were about five months old. We were out a lot so they often fell asleep in the car or their pram. I didn't know when they were tired – they'd just fall asleep anywhere, including under the play gym. If we were home I'd usually pick them up and pop them into bed where they would sleep more soundly. At about five months I could see the signs of tiredness like rubbing their eyes or getting noticeably grizzly. I'd stroke their foreheads after popping them in their cots. They'd turn their heads and then settle themselves to sleep.

We had a regular bedtime routine at night; dinner, bath, changing into pyjamas, a dark and quiet breastfeed then we'd carry them down the hall and into their cot. They associated this pattern with going to sleep. Soon they also established a regular three-sleeps-a-day routine and I always put them to bed at the same time. I really appreciated that baby-free time.

I found it harder as they got older and their sleep patterns changed. I got upset when they screamed instead of having their 9.30 a.m. sleep. When was I going to get anything done? It was worse when one slept while the other screamed. They rarely slept longer than one hour during day sleeps.

I learnt not to plan to do anything other than look after my babies, then if they didn't sleep I wouldn't get angry and upset. This mental adjustment was a big relief. I gave myself permission to do nothing but look after them. Anything else was a bonus. From around eight months the girls slept for 12 hours overnight. They also had two sleeps during the day. Occasionally they're unsettled if they're sick. When only one baby is unsettled, the other is rarely disturbed. They still have their dummies, just for bed and this is their main association with sleep. When I pop their dummies in, their heads magically flop on my shoulder. We continue to be firm when they have the occasional whinge at sleep time. We might go in and re-settle them up to two times but then just leave them to it. They might cry for ten minutes, then they remember that crying isn't going to make us go in there, so they lie down and we have a glass of wine!

Louise: Sleep is all new parents ever talk about. Like all first-time parents who hadn't had much to do with babies, I didn't have a clue. Twins magnify the sleep issues – at least with one baby you can lie down and get some rest when they sleep but with two they may never sleep at once, leaving you with no sleep at all.

Decent sleep was crucial for our happiness and survival but it took us months to find it. At first I couldn't tell when my babies were tired – they were probably desperate to be left alone for some sleep. Whenever a baby murmured I'd run in and pick her up, even though the poor thing was probably just rolling over. I must have driven them nuts and taught them how to be disrupted. Once we all learnt how to get the sleep we needed, we began to see a much brighter future.

When I was pregnant I didn't make any plans for where or when the babies would sleep. I thought when I walked in the door with them it would all fall into place. We had a cot set up in our bedroom but I wasn't sure they'd be in it straightaway, it seemed so big. We had two little soft sleeping bags, maybe they'd sleep in them. Or perhaps they'd sleep with us.

During the day I expected them to nod off and 'sleep like babies' until they were refreshed and ready to feed. I expected them to do the same at night. I had no idea how much sleep newborn babies need or how to tell if they were tired.

We were living in a two-bedroom house with Tony and me in one room and Tony's son, Eliot, sleeping in the other. At first we decided to put one cot with two babies in it in our bedroom. The girls breathed loudly, coughed and snorted all night. Babies are noisy. I was constantly listening for their next sound, so I couldn't sleep properly even when I had the chance. We disturbed them when we went to bed or got up to go to the loo, and couldn't have a lamp on to read. It also made it impossible to sneak in for a rest when they were sleeping during the day. Our household sleeping arrangements had become really haphazard by this stage, there was no routine and we were playing musical beds every night. No one ended up in the same bed they'd started out in. That lasted three nights. I was very confused. It was time for the sleep school. My local doctor was able to book me in to a mother and baby unit where twin mums go straight to the head of the queue.

After three months of chaos I was given eight magical nights of drug-induced sleep. The nurses bottle-fed the girls overnight while I slept. They promised to make sure the girls wouldn't die overnight. It wasn't just me that was overtired, the girls were exhausted too. I realised I hadn't been letting them get their sleep. They were tired and grumpy. They needed help to break their bad habits and learn how to sleep properly. The staff showed me how to get the girls to sleep at the same time. I stood in the room with them, comforting them until they seemed ready to fall off to sleep but not getting them out of bed. I rubbed their backs or foreheads to relax them then snuck out and then they'd drift off to sleep. Either one or both would wake between two minutes and half an hour later and I'd go back in and comfort them again. This went on day after day but I kept a record so I could see that things were gradually improving. They were sleeping for longer periods each day.

The big difference with twins is that they can both cry at once. In these circumstances one plus one does not equal two but about ten. Ten times as stressful and ten times as difficult to manage. When I had one in my arms and the other was yelling I felt inadequate. It took me a long time to accept that with twins there were times when I just couldn't do it.

By the time I went home, the girls were waking for a feed at 10 p.m. then stirring a few times but staying in their cots and mainly sleeping till early morning. This was brilliant. Sometimes when a dummy fell out they'd wake and cry wanting it put back in. I'd sneak in, pop it back and they'd float off again. This was happening regularly at first then the more sleep they got, the less violently they'd suck on their dummy and the less often it would fall out.

The best thing about having learnt a bit about how babies sleep was that I now knew what to do. I wasn't confused and could see a time when they'd sleep through the night (and so would I).

The girls shared a cot with their heads to the centre until they started to kick themselves off the backboard and bang heads waking each other. It was definitely time to start thinking about a second cot. It was also time to move the cots into Eliot's bedroom. He was 16 years old and slept through anything.

Once the girls began to sleep all night, they continued to just get better and better at it until a bout of illness threw routines into chaos. To a certain degree we started again after sicknesses when we got up to them all night, but they tended to have a good memory and fall fairly quickly back into their good sleep habits when they were well again.

These days, now that we all have a good grip on sleep, I'm a bit slack when the girls wake me at night. I jump into the cot of who ever is upset (they're big cots) and within minutes they're saying, 'Hop up, Mummy'. At first I thought they wanted to hop up, then realised they wanted me out so they could get some sleep!

Sleeping like a baby

When it's not working the way we'd like, sleep can become an obsession for parents of babies and young children. When there are two babies not sleeping well, you can end up with two tired, whingeing babies and two very exhausted, frustrated parents. It's complicated further if you have older children who are not sleeping well either.

Some babies, like some adults, sleep like logs through noise, chaos and disruptions, while others are very sensitive to their environment and easily disturbed.

Getting older children and toddlers into a pattern that will suit the whole family a few months before the babies arrive can help you feel more confident about getting the new babies into a routine too. Switching bedrooms, moving from cots to beds or learning to sleep without you can be done before you arrive home with the babies rather than all at once.

If your babies are settled and sleep well from the start you may never need to try 'comfort settling' techniques. Most babies can learn the difference between day and night and can properly learn to sleep solidly by day and by night. If your babies have a routine, if they associate particular things with sleeping, and get the sleep they need, they will probably get into good habits fairly quickly, and those busy early months might be a lot more enjoyable. The theory for getting twins into a healthy sleeping pattern is the same as for one child. The main differences are that it can be (much) harder when two babies need settling overnight, or if they wake each other crying, or are not in the same routine. Most, but not all, parents of twins wake the second baby to feed with the first and encourage the same feeding-sleeping routine.

> ANOTHER MUM SAYS   'With our first child we didn't have a full night of sleep for over three years. We got into the habit of letting him come into our bed at around midnight every night. This didn't change until I found out I was having twins and put my foot down. I was terrified that twins meant I'd be completely exhausted so I devised a sleeping plan. I started in hospital, refusing to let people visit when the babies were sleeping. When we came home from hospital I loved the routine as it gave me time to relax when I knew they'd sleep. I found life easier with the twins plus one than I did with my first little one. Twins made me do it right. I was busy but in control, and I was getting enough sleep to enjoy my family.'

How sleep works

Sleep is essential to health and happiness for babies and adults. We have cycles of light and deep sleep. So do babies. Small babies have cycles that go for between 20 and 40 minutes. Older children have cycles that last about an hour.

During the light sleep phases, we wake briefly and resettle ourselves. Babies do this, too, so if you resist running in to whip your babies out of bed when you hear a little squawk, they may resettle. If they're picked up out of bed every time they get to a light sleep patch, they may learn how to wake fully every time rather than resettling themselves back to sleep.

How can you tell if your babies are tired?

Tired newborn babies can just seem tired or they may frown, stare, grizzle, suck, yawn and sometimes have jerky movements. Signs of tiredness in older babies are whingeing or grizzling more, breathing loudly through their noses, wanting you to hold them constantly, rubbing their eyes and pulling their ears. They get bored, can't concentrate and can become clumsy, too. The longer you leave tired babies awake, the harder they will find it to get to sleep.

To wrap or not to wrap?

Many babies like the secure feeling of being firmly wrapped in a piece of material. It stops their reflexes from jolting them awake. You can wrap with a bassinet sheet or a stretchy bunny rug in winter and use muslin in warmer weather. The wrap shouldn't be too tight or they might feel restricted. The baby's head should not be covered. A baby that doesn't like being wrapped can just be tucked in with a tight sheet. This can decrease the impact of their startle reflexes and can keep them feeling secure.

It can be an adjustment for parents when the time comes for your babies to stop being wrapped. It can be done by gradually loosening the wrapping over a week or two. It may not bother them at all, or it may mean an unsettled patch that takes some adjustment. Being consistent with everything else associated with sleeping will probably hasten the adjustment.

Two washing baskets or share the bottom drawer?

Should twins go straight to cots or sleep in bassinettes first? It's up to you. Should they share a cot or have one each? Sudden Infant Death Syndrome (SIDS Australia) recommends if sharing a cot, have the babies' feet up either end. Once your babies start to move around the cot independently, put your twins to sleep in separate cots to reduce the risk of SIDS.

Reducing the risk of SIDS

SIDS is short for Sudden Infant Death Syndrome (SIDS) and used to be called cot death. It means the sudden, unexpected death of a baby from no known cause. SIDS is the most common cause of death in babies between one month and one year in age. Most babies who die of SIDS are under six months old.

Even though the cause is not known, you can reduce the risk. It's natural to be concerned about SIDS but if you're obsessing, talk to your maternal child health nurse or phone the SIDS office in your area.

- Put your babies on their backs to sleep.
- Sleep your babies with their faces uncovered.
- Keep your baby in a smoke-free environment before and after birth.
- Make your babies' cot up so their feet are close to the backboard.
- Use a firm, clean, well-fitting mattress.
- Do not put your babies on a waterbed or beanbag.
- Tuck in your babies' bedclothes securely.
- Quilts, doonas, duvets, pillows, soft toys and cot bumpers in the cot are not recommended.
- Becoming too hot or too cold may be associated with SIDS.
- There is increased risk of SIDS when babies less than four months old bedshare with someone who smokes.

Sleeping with your babies

If you've had one or both of your babies in bed with you, at around three months you need to consider whether you want to go on having them in your bed for a few more years. They can be moved to a cot and settled at three months but if left much longer, they won't be happy to change their sleeping situation. Children rarely choose to move from their parents' bed into their own until they are between three and five years old.

ADVANTAGES TO HAVING ONE OR BOTH IN YOUR BED

- They might cry less.
- You may have less night-time disturbances.
- You can breastfeed them without getting up.
- Some parents sleep better with their children close by.
- At least one parent will have an early night each night.

DISADVANTAGES TO HAVING ONE OR BOTH IN YOUR BED

- You all disturb each other, and babies are much noisier than they look.
- You may be half-awake all night worrying about rolling on your babies.
- There's no easy way of going back. They will probably want to sleep with you until they're at least three years old.
- They need you to go to bed when they do.
- Four bodies in one bed may feel quite crowded.
- You may feel you never have any physical space to yourself.
- Older children may feel very left out.
- You may have no quiet time together as a couple.
- It may be difficult to use a baby-sitter.

BED-SHARING CAN BE UNSAFE

Your babies may be at risk if they bed-share with someone who has consumed alcohol, taken drugs or is experiencing fatigue. If you sleep with your babies, make sure that their faces cannot become covered by bedding and keep them away from pillows. Use lightweight blankets rather than doonas or duvets. Place your babies in a position where there is no risk of them falling out of bed.

Ready for beddy?

If you're not sure about how to put your newborn babies down to bed, try following this pattern.

- Make sure they have a full tummy and a clean nappy.
- Wind down before bed, sitting quietly with your babies, talking to them soothingly or singing a lullaby.
- You may choose to wrap your babies.
- Dress them in the right gear for the weather, making sure they're comfy and clean.
- The room should be fairly dark, quiet, warm and comfortable, but not hot. Put your babies into their cots or bassinettes, say good night and don't look back. Leave the room quietly.

Associations – both good and bad

If you follow a regular routine, it helps your babies learn when it is time to sleep. You are doing them (and yourselves) a favour if they start to associate particular actions or changes with sleep time.

ANOTHER MUM SAYS   'On the way to bed we say 'nigh-nigh' to the funny potato man, to daddy's pictures, put their dummies in their mouths and kiss them goodnight while they're being tucked into their cots. This routine has been the same every night of their lives. Once they could talk they'd say 'nigh-nigh' to the plates and pictures themselves.'

USUALLY GOOD ONES
- Being wrapped or swaddled can make a baby think of sleep.
- A special toy can be given for bedtime.
- Dummies can be used for sleep only, so become associated with going to bed. If the dummy falls out, the baby may wake and cry, and need the dummy put back in before they can fall back to sleep.
- A breastfeed or bottle-feed before sleep, then being put into a cot awake usually works OK, but if they always nod off while feeding, you can have the same problem of a baby waking up and wanting a feed to get back to sleep.

POSSIBLY BAD ONES
- A parent staying in the room while the babies fall asleep may mean they feel they need you there to get to sleep.
- Many babies start life sleeping after a feed because the feed has exhausted them. Continuing to breastfeed them to sleep can mean they associate this comfort with sleep every time they're going down, and need it to go back to sleep after waking in the night.
- Being cuddled to sleep before being put in their cots can mean the babies may be unable to put themselves to sleep and may wake from a light sleep phase wanting you to cuddle them back to sleep again.

Dummies or no dummies?
The problem with dummies and sleep is that your babies may associate sucking them with actually falling asleep, then when the dummy falls out overnight, your babies may wake.

TIPS FOR GETTING RID OF THE DUMMIES

- If your babies only use dummies for sleeping, they need to learn to fall asleep without them. Put them down without the dummies and use comforting techniques to help them settle.
- If they use dummies through the day too, then you may need to cut down gradually on daytime use first. They might cry more during the day until they get used to not having it.
- Just decide it's over, get rid of them and forget it. The children will forget too before long, if you're prepared to weather the temporary storm.
- If they're around three years old, giving them to Santa, the Easter Bunny or trading them in at the toy shop for something fabulous works well, although you may still have a couple of hellish nights. Make sure there are no more dummies available.

IF YOU DECIDE TO CONTINUE USING DUMMIES

- Accept that you will be getting up overnight for around nine months to replace the dummies (have a few spares handy).
- Pin dummies to ribbons on pyjamas so that one day they should be able to pop them back in themselves.
- Or just give them one chance every night – if it falls out, bad luck. By around 12 months they've usually mastered popping them back in themselves, until they knock it out of the cot ...

(ANOTHER MUM SAYS) 'The girls loved their dummies and therefore so did I. We preferred to get up and pop the dummy back in to spending lots of time using other settling techniques. It also helped keep them happy during unsettled times in the day and would sometimes give me an extra five minutes peace at feed time to get them into the house, dash to the loo and grab a drink. At 16 months they just had their dummies for sleeps and this was a useful sleep association. All praise to the dummy.'

Day and night are different

From day one you can help your babies learn the difference between day and night. When your babies wake at night, keep the lights dim and sound to a minimum. This encourages them to stay sleepy. Sometimes babies fall into having their long sleep during the day. This is the sleep we're aiming to have overnight. If you are consistent with your techniques for teaching day and night, you may avoid this problem.

If you are keeping the babies on the same routine, you may not notice when only one baby has day and night confused. If both are sleeping their long stretch in the day, try waking them a little earlier each day so they move their long sleep to a more appropriate time. You can work with your babies to move them gently into a routine that suits your family.

Some people believe that if they keep their babies awake in the day that they will sleep longer at night. This theory doesn't usually work. In fact, the better a baby sleeps in the day, the more likely he or she is to also sleep well at night.

Late feed

The 10 p.m. feed (sometimes called the rollover feed) is where you feed the babies while keeping them very sleepy. This is part of the process of getting them to have a nice long 11–12-hour sleep overnight. Both bottle-fed and breastfed babies need to be lifted out of their cots for feeding, but it's usually done very quietly in the dark. It is not appropriate to feed babies their bottles in their cots as it can contribute to developing ear infections.

> (ANOTHER DAD SAYS) 'We used top of the range nappies overnight so they didn't need changing. I loved being completely in charge of the rollover feed. I fed both babies at my own pace and it was one way I could take some responsibility for their care.'

The babies will drink less and less at their quiet late night feed. At some point you'll feel they don't need that feed and you won't go in and they'll be so used to staying sleepy at this time of day that they'll (ideally) sleep straight through.

Sleeping through

Technically, if your babies are sleeping all night and only feeding once around 10 p.m., they are now 'sleeping through'. There's a lot of discussion when you're a new mother about whether your babies are 'sleeping through' and you can feel as though your parenting skills are on trial.

Don't be concerned about comparisons, they are often exaggerated and are meaningless in the scheme of things and only serve to make you feel worse if you're already feeling tired.

How much sleep do babies need?

(ANOTHER MUM SAYS) 'We have a friend who worked for one of the main sleep and behavioural clinics. He spent one day with us, going through how much the boys should be sleeping, how to recognise tired signs, how to decrease stimulation and controlled settling techniques. That day changed our lives. We had to work at it, but we were very motivated and we have maintained excellent sleeping patterns since. If you have twins you need to have a plan for how much and when they should be sleeping and you have to be strict with them.'

Babies are all different and have different sleep needs. Your two babies may vary enormously in their temperament, their need for food and their need for sleep. This guide is for parents who want some idea of what to expect, and is a guide to the average baby. As your babies get older, they will probably feed less often, be more wakeful in the day, and the length of their overnight sleep will probably increase.

The first month
The average newborn baby sleeps for about 16 hours out of every 24. Newborns typically sleep for about two hours at a time, night and day, waking around every three hours for a feed. Try to limit their awake time to about an hour. The chart on page 251 is an example of a day in the first month of the life of newborn twins.

Try filling in your own chart to see what is happening and whether a pattern is emerging. There may be more of a pattern to their days than you realise.

At two months
At two months your babies will probably be more awake and alert during the day. This is usually a more chaotic month, so they may seem a bit crankier and all over the place than they were in that first month. Ideally,

THE FIRST MONTH

6.30 a.m.	Baby wakes, change his/her nappy. Gently wake and change the other one. Feed both babies together.
8 a.m.	Change nappies, put both babies back to bed.
10 a.m. 11.30 a.m.	This routine is repeated.
1.30 p.m. 3.00 p.m.	This routine is repeated.
5 p.m. 6.30 p.m.	This routine is repeated.
9.30 p.m.	Feed and straight back to bed.
2 a.m.	Feed and straight back to bed.
6.30 a.m.	Start again.

they'll be having between eight and nine hours interrupted sleep overnight. They will wake to feed and then go straight back to sleep. They will have three daytime sleeps of about two and a half hours each. Their awake time should be up to about one hour and fifteen minutes between each sleep.

At three months
Typical three-month-old babies sleep for about ten hours overnight and have three daytime sleeps. Don't be disappointed if this is not what your babies are doing. If you can recognise when they're tired and are providing a warm, quiet, dark, comfy room and are patting and rocking them but not getting them out of bed when they're unsettled, that's all you can do.

On the next page is a flexible guideline for a day in the life of three-month-old babies. If your babies were born at 36 weeks or earlier they may not be ready for a three-month-old pattern yet.

AT THREE MONTHS

6 a.m.	Baby wakes, change his/her nappy. Gently wake and change the other one. Feed both babies together.
8 a.m.	Put both babies back to bed.
10 a.m. 12 noon.	This routine is repeated.
2 p.m. 4 p.m.	This routine is repeated.
6 p.m. 8 p.m.	This routine is repeated.
10 p.m.	Quietly feed both babies, then put them straight back to bed.
6 a.m.	Start again.

At six months
A typical six-month-old baby needs 11 hours sleep overnight and two daytime sleeps that are between three and three and a half hours long. They may be starting to eat solids as well as having breast or bottle.

At nine months
Ideally, 11 hours overnight, two hours sleep in the morning and one hours sleep in the afternoon, making a total of 14 hours.

At twelve months
A typical one-year-old sleeps for between 11 and 12 hours overnight and ideally has a morning and an afternoon sleep. The morning sleep is often the longer one, about an hour and a half is great, and in the afternoon they often only sleep for around 45 minutes.

At 18 months

At this age it's terrific if your toddlers sleep between 11 and 12 hours overnight, and have two hours sleep during the day The daytime sleep is usually around lunchtime so they're up before 3.30 p.m. (that's if you want them in bed by 7.30 p.m.). Children who wake early tend to hang onto their two daytime sleeps for longer.

The idea of having fun rather than sleeping kicks it at around 18 months–2 years. You could put your twins in separate rooms. If you don't have a spare bedroom but want to separate them you could put one in your bedroom for daytime sleeps.

Leaving them in their own room for the hour or two, even when they don't sleep, can mean a break for you. Just shut the door and put your feet up. Quiet time is better than nothing and sometimes they may play for an hour then sleep for two after that! The flip side of twins sharing a room at this age is that they can wake early in the morning and, rather than crying out to you, they will play games, sing songs and entertain each other while you have a little extra dozing time.

At two years

Most two-year-olds sleep for between 11 and 12 hours overnight and for between one and two hours in the afternoon.

At three, four and five years

- Ideally, three-year-olds sleep for 11 hours overnight and nap for about an hour during the day.
- Four-year-olds can sleep for about 11.5 hours overnight but don't usually nap during the day.
- Five-year-old children can sleep for about 11 hours overnight and no longer nap during the day.

Unsettled babies

Most babies have an 'unsettled' period during the first three months where they seem to cry for a couple of hours each day for no apparent reason. 'Unsettled' is a fairly lame description for two inconsolable babies screaming their lungs out. It's actually very stressful and if you're going to squabble with your partner, this is when it will probably happen. It's usually at the same time each day and often in the early evening.

Often both babies are unsettled at the same time. Two babies crying and wanting to be held can be difficult for two parents. Dinner is made with one hand or not at all or one parent tries to comfort both. Being a single parent or having older children who are cranky and needing attention adds to the stress. Try to remember that it (only) lasts until the babies are around three months old. The crying is said to peak at about six weeks.

One baby always wakeful, the other always sleepy

If one baby seems very tired and the other quite wakeful, you could play with the more wakeful one before feeding, letting the other baby have a sleep-in until it's evidently time for a feed. There's also no reason to keep a sleepy baby up just because the other one is more wakeful. It's the feeding together and sleeping at least partly at the same time that most twin parents find important.

Comfort settling

'Comfort settling' is a term used to describe the practice of teaching your babies to settle themselves back to sleep without your help. It is also sometimes called 'controlled crying'. It means an end to tossing them into your bed so you can all get some sleep. It's often used by parents who feel desperate to change their babies' sleeping patterns.

TIPS FOR SETTLING BABIES

- Extra breastfeeds settle some babies. Don't give extra formula feeds, as they need the comfort not the food.
- Dummies can calm them.
- Warm baths settle others.
- Wind up or electric baby swings can rock some babies into a relaxed or sleepy state.
- Wearing the babies in baby slings may settle them and let you get something done at the same time.
- Pop them both in the pram and go for a walk while the dinner is being prepared, or while other children are being bathed and given some attention.
- Remember that babies die from shaking but not from screaming.

Some parents believe that comfort settling is wrong – they don't want to let their babies cry. If you believe it's wrong, it's best not to do it. Sometimes only one parent believes it's wrong. In this case, you'll have to discuss it together and make a decision.

If your babies were pre-term, you may be uncomfortable with comfort settling. Leaving babies to cry when they began life with a bit of a struggle, can be very difficult. Don't start to teach them to sleep this way unless you're sure it's what you want to do. That way, you won't stop and start, which only confuses the babies and you.

Most parents find every instinct in their body tells them to pick up and comfort a crying baby, while the theory is telling them not too. Be prepared for these conflicting feelings by thinking about and planning when you'll start the process rather than beginning on a whim.

Before you begin

- Both partners need to agree to the plan. If both babies are unsettled, it'll be easier if you spend at least the first night settling one baby each.
- You both need to be determined and committed.
- Decide when you'll begin and talk about how you'll cope with the stress and frustration.
- If possible, arrange some help over those days so you can snatch some sleep.
- If only one of your babies is having trouble sleeping, move the settled baby into another room while you teach the other to sleep.
- Have earplugs or headphones and music handy.
- Have two charts drawn up and pencils handy to jot down the amount of time you spend settling each baby. This helps you see the progress you're making.

What to do

The guidelines below apply to babies less than six months old. The process is different for babies older than six months.

- Choose a time to start when you can cope with being tired the next day. You can start this any time in the day. It may be better to start after you've had some sleep.
- Make sure babies are clean, relaxed and not hungry.
- Put them to bed quietly at the appropriate time, say good night and leave the room.

- If the babies go to sleep, great!
- If the babies start crying, wait 30 seconds.
- If one baby is still crying after 30 seconds, one of you should go in. If both babies are crying, both of you go in quietly. If you're alone, choose which baby you'll settle first. Leave the light off. Try not to speak to each other – if you have to, then whisper.
- Don't pick up the crying baby. Rewrap him/her in the cot, if necessary.
- Pat, stroke or rock the baby gently till they settle.
- Leave the room before he/she falls asleep, unless you are alone and have another baby to settle.
- If so, switch to the other baby and begin settling, using the same techniques.
- When the baby is quiet leave the room, unless the other baby is crying.
- If crying begins, wait 30 seconds, then start again.
- Limit how long you do the settling for to about half an hour. If it's not working, get the baby/babies up again and have a break. Wait for their tired signs and you'll feel more refreshed about trying it again.
- You can vary your techniques, but don't change too often. Try rocking the cot, playing quiet soothing music, firmly placing your hand on her shoulder or gently stroking her forehead.
- Write down how much time is spent settling each baby so you can watch improvement the next day.
- Be consistent and use the same techniques for the babies that night and the following day.

What actually happens

The truth is it'll probably be very crowded and chaotic in there with two crying babies and two tired, on edge, guilty parents. You may not get much sleep that first night. Teaching babies to sleep pushes even the most reasonable parents to cross words and snide remarks. The worst part is, you've got another night of it ahead . . .

- Remember neither of you is enjoying this, so try to be reasonable.
- Think about how fabulous your lives will be when the whole household sleeps well every night.
- The more consistent you are, the faster they'll get the message. Keep in mind that tired babies aren't happy babies.

- It is confusing when both babies need attention. Most parents of twins feel the first night is a complete debacle. Most parents at some point feel frustrated and angry with the situation.
- Write down what's happening, otherwise you may think things aren't improving.
- You will probably succeed within a few days if you stick with the drill.

While you are settling babies, it can be reassuring to watch the clock or count the time it is taking in your head. When a baby is crying it can feel like hours, but it may only be minutes.

What to do for babies older than six months

ANOTHER MUM SAYS   'I wondered if all the going in and out was for the 'comfort' of the parents rather than the babies. In the end I put in my earplugs, took my sleeping bag to the other end of the house and shut every door in between. I don't know what they did that night, I just knew that as a single parent of twins I'd run out of options. The next night they slept for 11 hours, only waking once. I haven't looked back. We're all a lot happier now that we're sleeping properly and I don't think I did any permanent damage that night.'

It is easier to teach a baby to sleep when they are younger. Teaching babies older than six months to sleep doesn't involve being in the room with them all the time. Instead, the process requires you to comfort the babies for 2–10 minutes then leave them for 2–10 minutes.

- It's best to have two adults to deal with two babies. If you're a single parent, find someone to help you for a couple of nights.
- Check the babies are relaxed, warm, clean and not hungry, settle them on their backs in their cots.
- Say goodnight and leave the room.
- If they go to sleep, excellent!
- If one cries, wait 30 seconds, then one of you go in and settle the crying baby for two minutes. If they both cry, wait 30 seconds, then go in and settle using one settling technique (pat bottoms, rock, rub foreheads or backs).
- Leave as soon as they're settled or leave the room after 10 minutes, regardless of what state they're in.

- If either or both are still crying or have started up again in two minutes, return and settle using the same or another settling technique.
- Leave when they're settled or in 10 minutes, whichever comes first.
- If either or both are still crying in four minutes, return and settle.
- Leave when they're settled or in 10 minutes, whichever comes first.
- If either or both are still crying in six minutes, return and settle.
- Leave when they're quiet or in 10 minutes, whichever comes first.
- If either or both are still crying in eight minutes, return and settle.
- Leave when they're quiet or in 10 minutes, whichever comes first.
- If either or both are still crying in 10 minutes, return and settle.
- Leave when they're quiet or in 10 minutes, whichever comes first
- Keep going in every 10 minutes, leaving when they settle or in 10 minutes, whichever comes first.

Limit how long you do each period of settling to about half an hour. If it's not working, you don't have to persist. Have a break and get the babies up, give them a reassuring cuddle but don't take them out of the room. Stay by the cot so they get the message that they're not going anywhere. Avoid eye contact or encouraging behaviour. When they settle, place them back in their cots and try again.

What actually happens
It's hard but it will probably be worth it.
- You may feel frustrated by your babies' refusal to sleep.
- You may get angry with your partner.
- Thirty seconds can feel like an hour and two minutes can feel like forever.
- The first night may be close to unbearable so you may not feel like persisting into the second night.
- The second night may feel worse than the first but if you jot down what's happening, you'll probably see that your babies are already settling more quickly.
- It's tempting to revise your plans in the middle of the night. This is not usually a good idea, regardless of how sensible it may seem at the time.

- Babies at this age are very fast learners, and you'll probably have 12 hours sleep in a few nights time.
- The more consistent you are, the quicker they'll get the message.
- Remember tired babies and parents are miserable babies and parents.

What to do for children over a year old

For children older than one year, the process for teaching them to sleep is the same as for babies over six months.

- Don't give them opportunities to argue, just gently tell them they're going to bed and start the bedtime ritual.
- If they get out of bed, tell them next time you'll close the door, then next time close the door.
- If they're playing in their cots, you can go in and tell them to 'go to sleep' every ten minutes. Twins sharing a room may laugh at you, don't encourage them by laughing back.
- After one or two warnings you may choose to ignore them and leave them to it.
- Sleep patterns change as they grow older. If they're not going to sleep at their usual morning nap they may be cutting back to one daytime nap.
- Consider separating them if you have another bedroom. A twin sharing a room with an older sibling is worth considering.
- Consider putting one into your bed for daytime sleeps.
- If they vomit, clean it up then continue where you left off.

(ANOTHER MUM SAYS) 'The first few weeks at home with our newborn twins were fairly 'normal' in terms of a consistent feeding/sleeping pattern. It wasn't until several weeks later that a dreaded change began to emerge; the twins started to refuse to settle after feeds during the night. The most exhausting aspect of this was that they seemed to be taking turns so that there was no let-up. As they shared a room, it was impossible to do any form of controlled comforting. The baby whose turn it was would scream the house down, waking the sleeping baby in no time. We would then have two hysterical babies to deal with. When I was pregnant with the twins it had never occurred to me that we might put them in separate rooms. I had a sofa in their room to breastfeed them without having to move around the house with them. After resisting the need to separate them for months, I finally caved in. They were very light sleepers and obviously could not deal with each other's crying. As they got bigger they were too aware of our comings and goings and often woke as we were trying to remove the 'troublemaker' who had started to whimper. The only spare space we could find was our walk-in robe. While one twin slept in the luxury of a designer nursery, the other slept amongst the coats and handbags. Our family used to joke that she would probably grow up with a fetish for clothes. Separating our twins was not the complete answer to our problems, although it did reduce the stress associated with the twins waking each other.'

Illness

A bout of sickness can throw good sleeping habits out the window. They can stay out the window once the sickness has gone. All you can do is start to get your children back in to their old routine again. This is yet another area where it's difficult with twins. One gets sick, gets out of whack then the other gets sick and the situation is magnified.

You may decide to 'retrain' the one who is better, or you may wait until both are better before starting again. They often slip back into their good habits once you firmly remind them by sticking to the comfort settling technique.

From cots to beds

Depending on the detention capabilities of your cots, your twins may have schemed how to climb out by 18 months or earlier. At this point many parents decide it's time for beds to avoid accidents. The sense of adventure and the challenge of the leap can vanish once they are moved to beds. Pulling every book from the shelf, nappy from the box and piece of clothing from the cupboards should eventually lose its appeal too.

It can be a surprise the first morning they come pattering and laughing into your room and you realise you're still in bed so they've managed to jump the fence, usually by helping each other. If you can figure out how they're getting out and move any aids, they may last a few more days or weeks in captivity. If they haven't discovered how to get out themselves, then leaving them in their cots for as long as you can is very tempting.

ANOTHER DAD SAYS 'I'd keep them in cots till secondary school if they couldn't climb out.'

If a child gets out of the cot you need to make the room and surroundings as safe as possible.

- Don't leave heaters in the room or windows open.
- Have a night-light so wandering toddlers can at least see obstacles.
- Put a childproof gate on the door, although if they can climb the cot, they may also be able to climb the gate.

If your children are getting up because they really need you, go to them, rather than them feeling they need to come to you.

Return the toddler to bed with little attention and once settled, leave the room. Remind them that night-time is for sleeping and that's what you expect them to do. Letting them in your bed or providing lots of cuddles and attention will only encourage them to continue – work out if this is what you really want.

ANOTHER MUM SAYS 'It's tough, but being tough pays off when you all get your own space to sleep through the night.'

TIPS FOR MOVING FROM COTS TO BEDS

- Don't do it in the midst of other life-changing experiences for them, like the arrival of another baby, during toilet-training or weaning.
- Prepare them for the change, read storybooks on the theme and discuss that they will be doing the same soon.
- If you're shopping for new beds and new linen, involve them in the final choice. Narrow it down for them – this one or that one?
- If they're a bit tentative and there's room for cots and beds, let them share their room with their beds for a while to get comfortable with them before moving to sleeping in them.
- Some children sleep in the bed during the day and then the cot at night for a while.
- Cushion the fall with pillows or a quilt – they're unlikely to fall out but if they do they probably won't injure themselves, just get a fright.
- Some toddlers may be reluctant to change and start delaying bedtime. If you remain consistent, this won't last long.

Sleep schools

Capital cities have sleep schools, otherwise known as 'residential family services' or 'mother and baby units' to help families with sleep and sometimes other difficulties. Some of these are in the public system while others are private and are often attached to private hospitals.

Sleep schools usually use 'comfort settling' techniques to help you get your babies sleeping. Sleep school is not a last resort. Coming sooner rather than later can be helpful. You are not a failure if sleep patterns don't meet the ideal. Doing something constructive like booking into sleep school will help you get sleep sooner.

Many sleep schools try to function in a flexible family-friendly way. Most try to individualise the care available. Some can be more structured. This environment can be ideal for parents who feel things are out of control and for those who need support to find the strength and persistence to teach their babies to sleep. Your maternal child health nurse or GP can recommend and, where appropriate, refer you. See Resources, pages 340–47.

If you are a private patient, check with your health fund to make sure you meet the criteria for them to fund your stay. Take a note of the time and the name of the person you spoke to and ask them to put it in writing. The last thing a refreshed mother of twins needs is a surprise bill for thousands of dollars.

Some sleep schools offer day-stay for parents who just want to go in for a day for some help with settling their babies. Babies go too, and sleeping techniques are practised throughout the day. Parents learn how sleep works, are given information, advice and support. Residential stays, usually five nights, are for those parents who are exhausted or have very unsettled babies. There is often a waiting list but parents of twins frequently go to the top of the list. Most parents are so tired that staff will probably suggest sleeping for the first couple of nights, waking you for breastfeeds only, or not waking you at all if your babies are bottle-fed. They may even offer you a sleeping pill. During the day you'll be encouraged to rest in between settling and feeding your babies. After a couple of nights mothers are encouraged to get up when their babies wake and settle them with help from the night staff. This means you'll be confident when you go home.

The staff work in shifts, day and night, assisting you with settling your babies. You will have charts to fill in when each baby is asleep, feeding, awake or unsettled. A pattern emerges fairly quickly. Most parents leave feeling things have improved dramatically and with a sense of renewed confidence.

TIPS FOR SURVIVING SLEEPLESSNESS

- Get toddlers and older children into good sleeping habits before the babies arrive.
- Think about and prepare where your babies will sleep.
- Teach young babies the difference between day and night.
- Sleep when your babies sleep and don't worry if it's not at night.
- Routines help children establish good sleeping habits.
- If you say, 'It's bedtime', put the children to bed.
- Discourage stimulation and excitement before bed and at night.
- Seek help if nothing is working – you can't survive on no sleep for long.
- Keep in mind that this may be the most stressful time your relationship will face.

TIPS FOR PARTNERS

- Remember that teaching babies and children to sleep well is a job for both parents.
- It's in your interests to instil good sleeping habits in your babies – persevere, and you'll be having plenty of sleep at night.
- Decide on sleeping strategies together – when you're both tired, two heads are definitely better than one.

Coming, ready or not

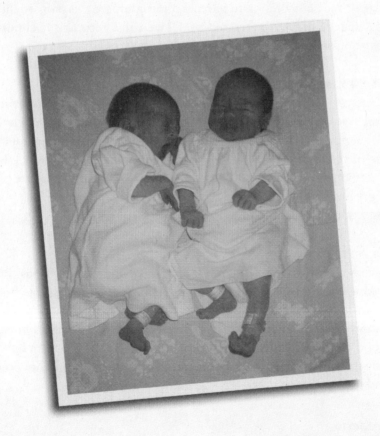

PRE-TERM BABIES

Pre-term babies

Pre-term babies are babies born earlier than the date they are expected. Many women successfully carry twins to term but twins do have a greater chance of being born pre-term. The average length of a twin pregnancy is 36 weeks. A pre-term baby is one born earlier than 36 weeks. It is better to be a twin born at 26 weeks than a singleton born at the same gestational age.

Continual improvements to hospital care and a better understanding of potential problems mean early help or treatment has greatly improved the prospects for pre-term babies.

Pre-term babies will often be referred to as having a 'corrected' age. This uses their due date as their 'corrected' age. A baby born at six months has three months development to catch up to a baby born at full term. Health professionals and parents often compare this baby to milestones achieved at their corrected age. This can continue for children until starting school.

Why it happens

Many factors are thought to contribute to pre-term labour of twins. They include an overdistended uterus triggering labour, the weight of the pregnancy on the cervix, dehydration, urinary tract infections or rupture of the amniotic sac, or it could just be that the pregnancy has decided to finish. Diabetes and heart disease are risk factors, as are placental problems, a previous pre-term labour, smoking, alcohol or poor nutrition, standing for too long and high levels of stress.

Why it matters

The earlier a baby is born, the more help he or she usually needs. Pre-term babies often need help breathing, feeding, keeping a stable body temperature and maintaining their sugar levels. Advances in medical technology now mean that most babies born after 24 weeks have a very good chance of surviving and thriving. Survival of pre-term babies depends on how healthy they are, how much they weigh, and how they respond to treatment.

Your reaction

Parents in this stressful situation react in many different ways. Some feel numb, others are angry, some don't want to know anything, others need to know everything. Many parents are in shock that their babies have arrived when they weren't expecting them for months. Most parents of pre-term babies are very upset. This is a healthy and normal way to feel.

Feeling out of control, numb, or like you are dreaming are also common reactions amongst parents who have tiny babies in special care. You may feel scared of your babies' size and fragility, and scared for them because they may die. Don't feel bad because you have these feelings. Talking with the hospital staff, the hospital social worker or a counsellor and parents of other babies can help you. In a very stressful and foreign experience it is quite normal to feel strange and upset. Some hospitals organise coffee mornings for parents of pre-term babies so they can share their feelings and experiences.

You may feel that something you did caused their early birth. Many women of very small babies go over and over the pregnancy, fearing they did or said something to cause it. Feeling jealous of those with bigger term bellies or with healthy, full term babies is also a natural response to your situation. Some mothers find it hard to be in the maternity ward or in the same room as mothers with full term babies.

If your babies are born early, they will have all their fingers, toes, fingernails, toenails and will be fully formed. They may be very sleepy and not able to suck, swallow and digest food yet. Often they won't be able to do these things until they reach their due date.

You may find you are shocked by your babies' physical appearance. They may be thin and wrinkled with downy hair all over them. Their heads may seem too big for their bodies, they may have spindly arms and legs. Often their chests are small and sunken, and can suck in with every breath. Many parents are very frightened by these tiny chests which they see working so hard. The sunken chests can also make the babies' tummies look large in comparison. Their skin can be so transparent that you see through to the red beneath, with their veins prominent beneath their skin and their thin little ears bendable because they haven't grown any cartilage yet. Some little boys testes haven't dropped and some little girls' clitorises can seem large and exposed. All of these very strange things are normal characteristics of pre-term babies because they haven't quite developed to the stage of full term newborns. They won't look different for long, because these characteristics will disappear as they get closer to their due date.

Some parents see their babies as tiny, vulnerable and beautiful, and all their protective instincts come flooding out. You may feel guilty if you're repulsed or terrified. Understand that you may feel angry, helpless, scared or sad. You may be experiencing grief over the loss of your pregnancy and the loss of two healthy bonnie babies. Anger with your partner, sadness, anxiety and guilt at not being able to protect them are all common responses.

ANOTHER MUM SAYS 'The first thing they said when I came round was, 'You have two little baby boys.' Mum had taken polaroids so I could see them. They were born at 27 weeks, and their feet were the same size as my thumb. When my older son was born, all we did was rejoice. With the twins, for the first 48 hours I panicked, I was trying to accept that they might not make it. I decided to pour every bit of love into these babies, and with that came confidence. Out of the 108 days the boys were in hospital, I was with them 107 days. I couldn't drive, everyday Dad or my aunty drove me to the hospital and home again. I had such a strong family base.'

ANOTHER MUM SAYS 'My boys were good weights but their good size didn't match their lung development and within ten hours a paediatrician and special care nurse appeared in my room announcing that they had significant Respiratory Distress Syndrome (immature lungs) and would be transferring to the NICU. It seemed like another world away. My first real visions of the boys were with them totally covered in tubes and respiratory equipment. This meant I could not see their faces and it really bothered me that I didn't know what my children looked like. They were also in opposite ends of the NICU room (I understood that this was so because the staff focused on providing one-on-one care). However, I wanted my babies side by side, thinking this would give them strength. I also felt torn being away from one when visiting the other. My boys' little lungs were heaving with the difficulty of breathing and my inability to act on my instincts to sweep them up in my arms and kiss and cuddle them, made me feel totally helpless. Their four days in NICU will remain in my memory for a long time.'

ANOTHER MUM SAYS   'I was really scared about seeing my babies and didn't really want to go. They pointed out that the babies were in bay seven, where they put the severest cases. I just didn't realise what a struggle it is to survive at that age. When I first saw them I felt the pressure to be maternal but I really didn't feel that overwhelming, warm feeling because they looked so sick. I didn't know what to do. There were lots of lights and machines and we didn't know if we were in the way or not. We weren't allowed to touch them because they were far too sick. Should I be in NICU or up in my room? The nurses were great and told me to do whatever I liked. But I didn't know what was expected of me. I didn't know if I was a bad mother if I spent two hours in my room. We spent ten minutes with them that first visit. Premmie babies are not like a normal babies, they really look like skinned frogs at that age. Their facial features aren't recognisable. They don't have any fat, they're pink. My boys were born at 800g and 600g. Their heads were the size of an orange, fitting easily into the palm of my hand; their body an ice-cream and icypole sticks for arms. I could put my rings on their arms. The only way I knew they were mine was they had the same hairline as their big brother and father.'

ANOTHER MUM SAYS   'My boys were born at 31 weeks. I was too scared to touch them and make them real. They were so fragile, I didn't know what was going to happen. I only named my boys after I held them to my skin. I realised then that if they died, I wanted them to die with a name.'

How your friends and family may react

Many parents feel angry with friends or family who don't respond in the way they want. They may not send flowers and presents. They may be unsure of what to do when your babies are fragile. They may not know whether you are celebrating. Others may be keen to celebrate while you are not ready. You may be holding off until you feel confident. It's not simple. You may want to let people know you would like their involvement by sending birth announcement cards or you could invite people to a christening or a naming ceremony.

(ANOTHER MUM SAYS)   'Tell your close friends and family what you need. I found it very isolating when people would tell me it would all be fine. They were denying my fears and the reality that it may not all be fine. I needed people to recognise how hard it was and be supportive and hopeful.'

Understanding what's going on

If you are worried about difficulties your babies are experiencing or disabilities your babies may have, ask the midwives and doctors, who will explain as much as they can. If you want to understand all the technical things the hospital is doing with your babies, ask and they will be explained. Write down any questions when you think of them. Keep asking questions until you feel you understand what you need to know. Writing down the answer may help if you are forgetting information at this stressful time.

Looking after yourself

It's physically and emotionally draining to give birth to twins but when they are in special care, the toll on your health can be much greater. Eating, sleeping, drinking water and resting are really important now.

If you're breastfeeding, it's very physically tiring. The exhaustion and stress can affect your milk production so it's in your babies' best interests that you rest and look after yourself as well as possible.

Care of pre-term babies

Neonatal Intensive Care Unit and the Special Care Nursery

Babies born before 33 weeks are likely to be in the Neonatal Intensive Care Unit (NICU) where there is one staff member for every baby. The babies need warmth as they don't have enough fat to keep themselves warm. Being kept warm artificially means they can use all their own energy to grow. They probably need help to eat and possibly to breathe as well. Staff in the NICU are highly trained to deal with your tiny babies and have a wealth of experience with pre-term babies so are a great resource.

You may be overwhelmed by the amount of machinery everywhere and the constant alarms and beeps surrounding your tiny babies. The babies are in incubators or open beds to give the doctors and nurses quick access to them. Most tiny premmies will have breathing equipment and breathing and heart rate monitors. They could also have blood pressure monitoring, drips in the umbilical cord or arms or legs and they may have oxygen monitoring.

The Special Care Nursery is for babies that are born at term but are sick and need some additional support. It is equipped to meet the needs of small babies, and staff provide a higher level of care than is available on the maternity ward.

These babies may be put into clear plastic boxes (called isolettes) with round holes in the sides. They provide a constant temperature for babies who need help to stay warm. Staff and parents can care for and touch the babies through the portholes.

These days it is common practice for hospital NICU and Special Care units to adjust the lights to parallel night and day. In most Australian and New Zealand nurseries the staff also try to handle and disrupt the babies as little as possible, using feed time to do most procedures. This seems to help babies to sleep more deeply and for longer periods, helping them to grow and get healthier. Although there are many noisy machines, the staff try to keep noise levels as low as possible, talking quietly.

You may find that you begin to notice what your babies seem to enjoy and what they find stressful. This can help you to make them more comfortable. Some parents find their babies like being sung to or having their foreheads rubbed, while others bring lambswool blankets in for their babies to lie on. You will need to wash your hands when entering the specialised areas, to help stop germs from the outside contacting the babies. The staff will show you the hand-washing practices.

(ANOTHER MUM SAYS) 'I felt tremendous pressure from some staff asking when I would and wouldn't be there. I couldn't be there all the time and felt disempowered from caring for my babies. I recommend putting a sign stating when you'll be there, so others don't keep asking your schedule.'

ANOTHER MUM SAYS   'We were never relaxed all the time that we had a baby in hospital. I felt on the edge all the time. The whole mental process of just being there is exhausting. Initially you don't know and you're just looking at all these things. Because we couldn't read the machines we'd read the nurses; watching their body language and their facial expressions. Then you soon work it out and it's sometimes more stressful to know. Like if there were a lot of nurses round the bed, you knew something was up. I could see one son's bed while walking down the corridor and when it was a hive of activity, I would prepare myself for the worst. Once it turned out the nurses were actually just coordinating each other's tea breaks. After losing my other son, sometimes there'd be three babies die in a day and we'd see them go into the little room and we knew what happened in that little room. We're instructed not to look at the beds with other babies. There's no privacy so you're not allowed to go up and look at them or ask the nurses about them. We knew when a baby crashed because of the alarm. I learnt to back off because I couldn't ride other people's wave as well. I used to sit there and knit – other mums would sing to their babies and chat with them but I really didn't know what to say and do. We held our two-year-old over the NICU crib saying, 'Here's your brother' and it really freaked him out. The alarms and monitors and everything were pretty scary for him to look at. He still had his normal routine and would come into hospital on the weekends. We were always in turmoil, we always wanted to be somewhere we weren't. When we were home, we'd want to be at the hospital and when at hospital we'd want to be home with our other son.'

Kangaroo care

Most nurseries in Australia and New Zealand use 'kangaroo care' for babies who are stable. Kangaroo care is skin-to-skin contact, usually between the mother's breasts or on the father's chest. Babies seem to respond to the memory of being back in the womb, hearing their mother's heartbeat and voice very close.

Research shows babies who have this contact cry less, sleep better, gain more weight, are more alert and have a better chance of breast-feeding successfully. It also helps stabilise their heart rate and breathing. Skin-to-skin contact gives the parents an opportunity to feel closer to their babies and feel more confident in caring for them.

ANOTHER MUM SAYS 'Two things that really helped my husband and I to bond with our babies were kangaroo cuddling and massage. I asked to kangaroo cuddle my boys and would suggest others do so, even if they are hooked up to machines. I asked the physiotherapist to show me how to massage the boys. I could rub their arms, back and legs with massage oil. She also taught me to recognise signs that they'd had enough. They would only tolerate a few minutes at a time but it really helped me to 'care' for them. I'd been robbed of that nurturing role and felt cuddles and massages really helped us all.'

ANOTHER MUM SAYS 'Alone in my hospital room upstairs I felt empty and cold. I walked past the rooms listening with envy to new baby cries. I missed my-two-year old and missed not being able to cuddle my babies. The boys were born at 34 weeks, and they went through many invasive tests. I was discouraged from handling them because they needed to rest so much. Despite the incredible dedication and wonderful skills of the doctors and nursing staff ... it didn't seem right. In retrospect, I wish I'd acted on my instincts and picked them up and cuddled them at length. It would have been the right thing for them and me.'

Pre-term twins sharing cots

Some hospitals and parents encourage sleeping pre-term twins together. Both babies need to be in a stable condition for them to share a cot. It may not be as simple as it sounds with all the tubes and wires involved. The benefits appear to be that the babies settle well, stay warmer and are quicker at learning to feed. They cry less, are less irritable and snuggle up to each other.

Feeding pre-term babies

With pre-term twins, the circumstances are not perfect from the start. Some pre-term babies are not able to start breastfeeding immediately. Their digestive system may not be developed enough to digest food, so they may need to be fed intravenously. Their ability to suck isn't usually effective until around 34 weeks, when this reflex develops. For a pre-term baby sucking can take up more energy than the food provides. In these circumstances they may need to be fed intraveneously. Then on to tube-feeding which can be breastmilk via a tube. Before a baby can breastfeed, she or he must be able to suck, swallow and breathe without choking or turning blue.

ANOTHER MUM SAYS   'Once my babies arrived, breastfeeding seemed essential to me. They arrived seven weeks early and were in hospital for four weeks. Breastfeeding didn't come naturally and neither did expressing. I expressed for four weeks. I had no idea about breast pumps but found my local pharmacy hired them and were a lot more helpful than the hospital. The boys were fed my breastmilk through tubes every two then three hours for the first three weeks. From three weeks I began breastfeeding them once a day, then twice a day after that. I had only fully breastfed them for 24 hours before they left hospital. I look back now and realise I needed more help with feeding when I first arrived home. Being pre-term meant they tired more easily, so initially the feeds were more frequent. I needed to change their nappies during the feed to wake them up again. I also gave them a bottle rather than a breastfeed after a bath, as they were too sleepy to suck. I breastfed them until they were nine months old. I thought it was really important that they received breastmilk with antibodies. Breastfeeding was easier than bottle-feeding in the long term. My boys had absolutely no head or neck control for months. I found I could support them more easily in my arms when breastfeeding than I could when bottle-feeding. There was a lot of trial and error and lack of sleep but I'm glad I persisted, it was really rewarding.'

Try not to be discouraged if your babies can't go to the breast immediately. There are many women who successfully establish breastfeeding after months of expressing. Don't be discouraged if the amount of breastmilk you are expressing seems low, it's a common reaction, and once your babies do the sucking your supply will be stimulated and you will produce more milk.

By starting to express breastmilk immediately, you can establish your supply, providing breastmilk for feeds and preparing for when your babies are ready to suckle. If your babies are born early, nature does its best by filling your breasts with pre-term breastmilk, which has a higher fat, protein and mineral content.

Providing breastmilk can have an enormous positive effect on both you and your babies. You are the only one who can provide this perfect source of nutrition and it's an excellent way to feel you are very involved in your babies' care. Many mothers of twins in NICU and the Special Care Nursery say expressing breastmilk gave them a sense of purpose and involvement in the lives of their babies.

If your babies are very pre-term and are not ready to be tube-fed breast milk, you can express your milk, which will start the supply-and-demand cycle. You can freeze this expressed milk for the babies to be given when they're ready for breastmilk.

Expressing

ANOTHER MUM SAYS 'I decided to breastfeed my premmie boys, so moved into the world of expressing and freezing milk. I did not start actually breastfeeding the boys until they were a month old. It was difficult waking up at 4 a.m. with these huge leaky breasts and no one to feed. I hired a machine. In retrospect, I really needed help with this and should have contacted the Australian Breastfeeding Association.'

Start expressing as soon as you can after the birth and within 24 hours. The midwives or breastfeeding consultant will help you. A small amount of colostrum is of enormous benefit to your babies. If there's a delay because you have been ill, you can probably still breastfeed. If you're very weak or still unwell, ask the nurses or your partner to express your milk for you. If you are expressing, shorter, frequent sessions are better for your milk supply and gentler on your nipples

If one baby is weaker or sicker than the other, you may decide to give her or him all the colostrum or breast milk if your supply is low at the start. Or you may decide to divide it. If you can breastfeed one baby, then try to express from the other breast while feeding. This will make the expressing more effective, as the stimulation on the other nipple helps promote the let-down.

ANOTHER MUM SAYS 'Because I had premmies I was under a lot of pressure to breastfeed when I really hadn't planned to. When the midwives came at 3 a.m. to wake me and squeeze my breasts I thought, 'Who are these parasites?' Two mls came out and I thought that was so few and I only learned later how valuable that small amount is.'

HOW TO EXPRESS

You can express by hand or with a manual pump or an electric pump. Pumps should be available through the hospital but can also be hired from the La Leche League New Zealand or the Australian Breastfeeding Association. Both also have detailed pamphlets and counsellors to advise you on expressing. Your twin club may hire out breast pumps and many chemists and baby stores sell them. The sort of pump you use depends on how often you intend to express. If it's occasionally then you may choose to express by hand, if it's all the time, then you may buy an electric pump. You can get double pumps that express both breasts at once.

Nipple stimulation is what causes the release of hormones for let-down and milk production. Nipple stimulation is usually better by hand than by pump because it mimics the way the babies suckle. The first drops from your breasts will be tiny amounts of colostrum. This colostrum will continue for the first few days after your birth. The drops are precious, providing nourishment and resistance to infection, so make sure your babies get them.

EXPRESSING BY HAND

- Have a sterilised bowl or container ready to catch your milk.
- Stroke your breast gently but firmly in the direction of the nipple.
- Using your other hand, squeeze your thumb and forefinger on opposite sides of the areola.
- Squeeze rhythmically and from the breast, not the nipple.
- Move your fingers around the areola to empty the milk reservoirs evenly.

EXPRESSING BY ELECTRIC PUMP

- Begin by stimulating the nipples and massaging the breast.
- Start and end on the low speed, and build the speed up if necessary to extract the milk.
- Express every 2–3 hours for five minutes one side, five the other and then repeat so it's about ten minutes total per side. To build up your supply, you may decide to express a bit longer.
- Have a decent five-hour break overnight to sleep.

(ANOTHER MUM SAYS) 'I pumped one breast at a time so I had a free hand to massage my breast. When expressing you need to be comfortable and have things close to hand, just as when you're breastfeeding. My husband wasn't sure what to do and I just asked him to keep me company and put the expressed milk in the bottles then the fridge. I expressed a bit longer than the breastfeeding consultant advised, in order to build up enough supply to feed two babies.'

Freezing and defrosting breastmilk

Breastmilk storage bags are available from chemists. These are expensive but useful and come with full instructions, sealing clips and date markers. You can also use new sandwich style plastic bags or sterilised plastic containers. Don't use glass containers, because they can destroy some of the milk's antibodies during reheating.

Breastmilk keeps for 48 hours in the fridge, or for up to three months in the freezer. Expressed breastmilk thaws very quickly. Place the container under a running tap and allow the water to gradually get warmer (not hot). It will defrost in less than a couple of minutes. Don't defrost breastmilk at room temperature or in the microwave because this can affect its quality.

Tube-feeding pre-term babies

Your babies may be fed your breastmilk through a fine plastic tube. The tube is passed through their nose or mouth into their stomachs and is usually left in so your babies feed regularly. Some babies are fed at intervals while other babies are on a constant drip.

Tube-feeding doesn't hurt or upset your babies but after a while they can start to resist it. They may be restless and suck on the tube or turn their heads while they're feeding. When this happens they seem ready for breast or bottle-feeds. They are usually introduced to one 'sucking' feed per day, then are slowly built up until the breast or bottle eventually replaces the tube.

If your babies are not able to have breastmilk yet

Some babies are too sick to have breastmilk or formula and are fed a highly nutritious substitute. This goes intravenously directly into the blood. Breastmilk and formula can only go to the gut. This substitute is a balance of glucose water with vitamins, nutrients and fats, which provide enough nutrition for the babies' bodies to function normally and for them to grow. If your babies are fed intraveneously you can still prepare to breastfeed them when they're ready by beginning to express your breastmilk and establishing your milk supply. You can freeze this expressed breastmilk to give to them later.

Colostrum is a fantastic way for premmie babies to start their milk feeds. The tiniest quantities contain concentrated amounts of nutrients and immune agents. Colostrum is the concentrated food your breasts produce before your breastmilk comes in. It has a natural laxative that helps get rid of the thick meconium and introduces the baby's tummy to 'digestion' in the gentlest possible way, because it is so much easier to digest than full breastmilk or formula. If your babies are being fed intraveneously, you can freeze your expressed colostrum for them to be fed first when they are ready.

Many women breastfeed their twins successfully after a very rough start. Try not to be discouraged by being unable to breastfeed your babies at the beginning, or if your supply seems low.

Keep in mind that:

- Breastmilk will give them the best possible start in difficult circumstances, and every drop counts.
- Short, frequent expressing sessions are easier and more helpful when building up your supply (5–10 minutes every 2–3 hours).
- Expressing near your babies or having a photo of them with you may help.
- Once your babies are breastfeeding, your supply of milk will build up to meet their demand.
- Most hospitals have highly trained breastfeeding consultants on staff.

As well as those in hospitals, there are many private breastfeeding consultants available. You could ask a midwife you trust or the Australian Breastfeeding Association or La Leche League in New Zealand to recommend someone.

The Australian Breastfeeding Association and the La Leche League (NZ) provide great support to mothers of pre-term twins and 24-hour phone counselling.

Bottle feeding your babies with either breastmilk or formula
Pre-term babies drinking from a bottle are usually feeding the same amount as full term babies by the time they leave hospital.

Some small and pre-term babies often do better with longer thinner teats to stimulate the sucking reflex. Some do better with a faster teat (one with more holes) as they don't need to suck as hard, while others find the milk comes out too fast and they can't control the flow. Positioning the babies correctly is very important. Their heads should be in line with their body as it is when in a breastfeeding position. Their chins shouldn't be down on their chest as they need to have the teat in the back of their mouth to suck properly.

Looking after pre-term babies

It may take time for you to learn or gain the confidence to care for your babies. Ask the staff what things you can do to help care for them, like changing nappies or helping with feeds.

Sick pre-term babies can be unsettled and tense and difficult to look after for a while. These babies can easily get out of breath or go blue if they get upset or even when they cry with hunger. This can be distressing and it's natural to feel nervous and to try not to let your babies cry for a single moment. A slight drop in your babies' oxygen levels can also increase their irritability and make things seem worse.

Pre-term babies can also adjust to the noise and lights of their hospital nursery so that when they get home the quiet may upset them. They might also be very sensitive to touch after sometimes months of drips, tubes, needles and examinations. They may seem intolerant of any handling, and even a gentle nappy change can distress them.

Talking about your babies and your experiences and feelings with your partner and any of the following people might be helpful:

- the 'follow up' nurse (most nurseries have one)
- other nursing staff
- parents of other babies in the unit
- AMBA and NZMBA pre-term babies contact
- hospital psychologists
- hospital social workers

You can also check websites for support groups.

Possible problems for pre-term twins

ANOTHER MUM SAYS 'If anything could have gone wrong with our surviving son it did. Each day there was a drama which didn't happen in 99 per cent of cases, but did in ours. It was always a roller-coaster ride. I remember saying, if he's not going to make it, let it be now. We'd be told he was stable. Most 26-week babies are ventilated with oxygen for three weeks but he was ventilated for four months. Babies that are ventilated often develop hernias because of the pressure downwards, so need a hernia operation. He had IVs in his head. The only thing that made him look less awful was his hair but they'd have to shave it to put the drugs in. The nurses said not to worry because it would grow back but it did upset me – his hair made him my baby. It was a battle, but he was winning. Once he opened his eyes, I fell in love with him. He recognised me straightaway. It was difficult for my husband. He still had to function at work and then come home and deal with a hysterical and emotional wreck. For me, it was important that he still had a drink after work on a Friday night for a couple of hours and have some time for himself.

Babies normally go down from bay seven to bay one. We went to bay six and left hospital from there. He always had his own nurse. We didn't have a normal premmie experience.'

ANOTHER MUM SAYS 'My babies were born at 33 weeks. For the first three days the boys weren't feeding much at all, their urine output was low and they had apnoea. It was a frightening world with bells and buzzers going off every second. It was hot and sterile and so hard because we couldn't hold our babies. Once over the first five days the boys were getting better and we were allowed to change nappies and have the occasional cuddle. We used to be so excited about a nappy change because it was contact – we're not excited by that any more.'

Breathing difficulties

A baby's lungs aren't usually fully developed until 34 weeks gestation. If your labour starts early, steroids may be given to you to help develop your babies' lungs before they are born. If steroids aren't given in time some babies have respiratory distress syndrome (RDS). Most early pre-term babies may still have a degree of RDS even with the steroids. These pre-term babies lack the fatty substance known as surfactant to stop the air sacs in their lungs from collapsing. They need help to breathe properly. If your baby is being treated for respiratory distress, a tube is put through their mouth or nose into the main airway that leads to the lungs and is connected to a ventilator, then the ventilator breathes for them. Over time their lungs will produce the surfactant needed to breathe without help.

The use of artificial surfactant gets these babies through the critical period. By school age most children born prematurely will have outgrown these problems.

Some pre-term babies have milder breathing problems where they can breathe without a ventilator but need more oxygen than is available in the air. They are given more oxygen through a hood or nasal prongs. A sensor is taped to your baby's tummy, back, toe or finger to measure the amount of oxygen in their body.

Heat loss

Pre-term babies can have difficulty controlling their own temperature, and can also lose heat very easily. They are usually looked after in temperature-controlled isolettes until they have enough fat and maturity to maintain their own temperature.

Sugar levels

Pre-term babies may not have the stores of glucose they need to maintain their sugar levels. They can also produce too much insulin, which works by decreasing blood sugar levels. They may need intravenous therapy or frequent feeds. The blood or urine might be checked regularly for sugar levels.

Lack of oxygen

Anoxia is a lack of oxygen to the brain and can be a common problem in very pre-term babies. It can cause death of brain tissue and result in bleeding to the brain. This may damage an unimportant or a small area and have no obvious effects on the brain, or it can be so bad that other vital organs are affected.

Low immunity

Because pre-term babies are born before they receive all their mother's immunities they are very susceptible to infection. Some antibodies cross the placenta but not enough to protect the babies against everything. Their ability to create their own antibodies doesn't kick in until later, sometimes up to three months old. The IV lines and other invasive procedures also make them more vulnerable to infection. This means hospital staff have to scrub thoroughly before and after handling your babies and the equipment, and you must too. Wear a mask if you have even a cold or a cold sore and tell nursing staff if you don't feel well.

Anaemia

Pre-term babies can have anaemia as their red blood cells break down quickly and they don't make lots of new ones. Iron supplements or a blood transfusion can be given if the anaemia is severe.

Jaundice

Jaundice is quite common when babies are full term and even more common when babies are born earlier. It makes your babies' skin look yellow and is caused by the high levels of bile pigments in the babies' blood and tissue. These bile pigments are a by-product of the process of breaking down red blood cells, when the babies can't efficiently excrete them and they build up in the body. About 50 per cent of babies are jaundiced in the first week of life. These are all watched closely and treated because in about one per cent of cases, jaundice can cause brain damage if not treated. Special lights directed on to the babies break down the bile pigments so the babies' livers can process them. In occasional severe cases, babies may need an exchange transfusion where blood is removed and replaced.

Apnoea

Apnoea is a common problem in pre-term babies, because their reflexes are immature and they 'forget' to breathe. A baby born at 30 weeks or earlier is more likely to have apnoea. When they stop breathing, their heart rate drops. The NICU has monitors on every baby and alarms sound if a baby's breathing and heart rate slow. The nurses attend to them immediately and gently tickle their feet or stroke their chest to start them breathing again. If they don't start breathing, the next step may be blowing some oxygen on their face or a bag and mask attached to oxygen may be put on their face. It's a very common situation that the nurses are very used to and practised in, but parents can feel helpless and very scared. Alarms, nurses running and a pale or blue baby can be very frightening at first but often parents who've been around for a while just step out of the way or even stimulate the baby themselves. A percentage of babies receive some medication to help stimulate their breathing and to counteract this problem. Your doctor will tell you if this happens.

Noises

Pre-term babies often make lots of grunting noises all day and night. The grunting is caused by the baby's attempt to create what is called a continuous positive airway pressure (CPAP). Pre-term babies' lungs tend to collapse completely after they exhale because of lack of maturity. Taking the next breath is hard work and babies get very tired and many eventually need some form of help. The grunting sound is made when the baby forces air out through a slightly closed pharynx. Their chest may sink in rather than rising because the chest muscles that would usually expand the chest aren't strong enough to do their job.

Immunising pre-term babies

Provided they are well, babies born pre-term should be immunised at the usual chronological age, beginning at two months after birth, without 'correcting' for prematurity. Pre-term infants have been shown to mount an adequate antibody response.

ANOTHER MUM SAYS   'Within three months of leaving hospital both the boys went back in with bronchiolitis (like baby asthma) one week after the other. Most of the babies on the children's ward were multiples. Prematurity increases the risk of contracting this and, being highly contagious, it is hard to avoid transfer to a twin or multiple. We were back to tube-feeding and oxygen, but I felt quite experienced in these areas and coped well. Being pre-term is a legacy they live with for the first couple of years of their life. I was told not to have the twins around sick children. I had a two-year-old that attended crèche so how could I avoid it? This just added to my feelings of guilt. Luckily, they recovered well from the bronchiolitis and have so far avoided any other major illnesses.'

If you are worried about whether one or both of your babies will survive, ask the doctors and nursing staff to explain the possible health outcomes. You may want to discuss your feelings, concerns and wishes and find out when the critical period is likely to be over.

Going home without your babies

ANOTHER MUM SAYS 'I came home two weeks before my babies. I cried the whole day I had to leave them in hospital. I would visit them twice a day for three hours each but all I could do was sit by their cribs and look at them. I continued to express milk but I felt useless. I was also torn because I had to leave my two-year-old behind and she didn't understand. She was cared for by my husband and family members during that time, which required a lot of co-ordination. In theory I thought this time at home without my babies should have helped my physical recovery but because that is so connected to emotional recovery, this didn't happen. The emotional cost of their 'tough' beginning was substantial. Their time in NICU and Special Care surely affected the natural bonding process that occurs. I felt frightened by my feelings and resentful of other people's ways of helping. I had a mothercraft nurse coming in to help the first week the boys were home. She took over the babies and I immediately realised this was preventing me from re-creating what I'd lost. I needed to be the one holding the bottles for their feeds and providing the hands-on care for the boys. Thankfully I identified this need and tried as delicately as I could to make this clear to people around me and changed my arrangements. Within a week I arranged for a young friend to come and help instead, who was an experienced baby-sitter but untrained in the ways of baby care. This was just perfect for me because I was able to direct her and take some control again.'

ANOTHER MUM SAYS 'The first night home without the boys was just terrible. I was just so upset by the whole ordeal and worried about leaving them at the hospital. We really did not feel that they were ours until they were home.'

If your babies are in Special Care you may be well enough to go home before they are. This can be distressing. Leaving your babies behind can tear at the bond you have with them and you may grieve for that physical proximity. Many parents find it difficult to leave the hospital but at the same time feel relieved.

Many mothers also grieve because they have lost the future they had imagined, arriving home from hospital with two healthy babies. The new life they saw themselves living has been whipped away.

Going home without your babies may also mean hard work with expressing milk day and night and travelling to and spending time at the hospital. The hospital will probably be happy for you to visit your babies whenever you like. Taking a photograph of your babies home with you might be comforting.

If you live some distance from the hospital or if you have other children to care for, you may not be able to visit your babies as often as you'd like. Phone the baby unit and talk to staff about how your little ones are progressing. The nursery never closes.

If you are reluctant to leave your babies, you could try insisting on staying in hospital. Let the staff know how you feel and see what can be arranged. Sometimes it's possible to stay at the Nurses Home or some other accommodation can be provided.

Sometimes one baby is ready to come home before the other. You may feel guilty about being with one baby while you feel the other also needs your attention. This is common with twins and you will probably never resolve this one, so the easiest solution might be to stop feeling guilty. They will always swap roles as far as who needs what, back and forth, each one needing more attention at different times – even if it seems impossible now, it will probably work out fairly even in the long run.

Some hospitals prefer to keep pre-term twins together in the nursery until the smaller or sicker one is also ready to leave. There is documented evidence that an unwell twin can thrive if their twin is placed in the crib with them. Some parents of twins agree with this policy, while others prefer to take the opportunity to ease their way into caring for their two new babies by taking one home. Some parents report having bonded with the baby they first take home, then resenting the intrusion of the other when they come home too. This is completely understandable and natural, but may be an additional pressure on you.

You might do what you can to all stay together until both babies can come home. If not, when it's time for both your babies to leave the hospital, you and your partner could spend a couple of nights in the hospital caring for your them. Many hospitals have an overnight stay room for this purpose. You may be nervous about taking such small babies home. Others have been in charge of looking after them and now you are. It is hard to leave the nursing staff behind. Remember, they are a phone call away day and night, so ring them for advice or reassurance.

TIPS FOR SURVIVING LIFE WITH PRE-TERM BABIES

- Remember, all of your feelings are normal.
- Talk to your partner about your feelings.
- Name your babies as soon as you feel ready.
- Ask questions of the staff caring for your babies.
- Ask if you can change your babies' nappies, bathe them and give them a massage.
- Talk and sing to your babies.
- Express to boost your production of breastmilk.
- Talk with others who have been through what you're going through.
- Your babies may appear fragile but try to treat them normally and encourage others to as well.
- Remember that premmies can be slower to reach milestones than full term babies. Be patient.

TIPS FOR PARTNERS

- Your partner may need an enormous amount of emotional support, she may be in shock because she was not expecting her babies to arrive for months.
- Look after yourself, talk to friends, family or counsellors about your doubts and worries.
- Talk with your partner and listen. You are not expected to have the answers, just listening is really helpful.
- Learn about breastfeeding and expressing breastmilk so you can support and encourage her.
- Many mothers of premmies start to talk about wanting to have another baby and 'get it right' straightaway. Don't panic, you can talk later.

When bad things happen

LOSING A TWIN

When parents lose a twin

Parents who lose both their twins suffer an obvious tragedy. When parents lose one of their twins, the loss is different from the loss of both twins or the loss of a single baby and is often underestimated. They lose both a precious baby and the special achievement in having twins. People can be ambivalent if 'only' one baby has died. Parents who grieve may be judged as failing to be grateful for the living one, especially if it's before the birth or in the first few days.

Loss of a baby in pregnancy

The loss of a baby during pregnancy is a traumatic experience. Parents never forget a baby who dies. The loss of one twin brings confused emotions if parents still have one baby to love whom they may also be scared of losing, and who reminds them constantly of the one they've lost.

A loss in later pregnancy

The loss of a baby at any stage has a significant and lifelong impact. If a twin dies in pregnancy, the pregnancy continues for the living twin. The baby will be in utero until the birth. It is impossible to imagine surviving the death of a baby without some outside help. When a twin dies, parents may have to live through well-meant but hurtful comments from those who say they should be happy to have one baby, or from those who deny that a death during pregnancy is actually the death of a much-loved baby. Often people don't know what to say and avoid dealing with the grief. Parents who have lost a baby in pregnancy may feel angry with their partner if they do not always seem to share the same feelings. People express grief differently. Their grief may be submerged while they are dealing with and looking after another living baby. They may also mourn their surviving twin's loss of companionship. It is very important for parents and family members to let themselves feel terrible.

Parents have reported a range of feelings including:

- disbelief, numbness, disappointment, emptiness, anger
- an inability to accept the death or to grieve adequately for the dead baby while facing the continuing pregnancy
- terror about the birth of the live baby
- fear of how the baby who died will look when born
- sadness at being seen as parents of one baby and no longer as parents of twins or more

- jealousy of other parents of healthy babies
- being constantly reminded of the dead baby by the surviving twin
- anger towards the baby for dying and for the loss of all their hopes and plans
- guilt over not being able to 'protect' the baby from dying
- difficulty bonding with the surviving twin
- anger towards others because of feelings of frustration
- guilt for having such thoughts
- wanting to know why it happened, and partners often feel they need to 'protect' the mother from further hurt

Loss of a baby at or around the birth.

Most parents continue to think of their single surviving twin as a twin even if the co-twin was stillborn, and they usually want other people to think this way too.

ANOTHER MUM SAYS 'One baby was doing a lot better than we thought. But the other baby's kidneys weren't working. We were told that he was in trouble and were asked for our opinion on whether or not to continue treatment. At first I didn't know what that meant. Once we had the medical advice we knew straight away that he wasn't going to make it. They said we could do this whenever we liked. We chose the following day, a time was worked out, and they asked if there was anyone else we'd like to come with us. We decided we'd like to be by ourselves. They rolled our baby into the room in a crib. He was beautifully dressed in clothes I learnt some ladies had knitted. They lifted me this tiny light baby and I just couldn't believe it was my baby. He looked black in colour. He was still breathing. His eyes were still fused so he couldn't open his eyes. We held our little bundle thinking, this is awful and tragic. I didn't know whether I'd know the moment when he died. Afterwards I realised that wasn't important. We were devastated but I knew it was the right thing. I couldn't ask this little baby to keep living. We spent a couple of precious hours with him then we sat in our room in stunned disbelief. Our baby stayed in the hospital for a couple more days so that we could visit him when we wanted to. I didn't want him in my room because I knew I had to focus on my living baby. I don't have any regrets with the way we handled the death and time with him. I had to be there for my living baby and get on with essential tasks like expressing milk for him and being a mother to our other son. This limited the grieving process. My body went into shutdown mode. The rest of the world just went on without us and I really can't remember a lot about it. We also felt we couldn't celebrate the birth. Friends just don't know what to do. We wanted people to acknowledge the fact that we'd had two babies. Everyone gives you flowers because they don't know what to give you. I'd give people bottles of gin and boxes of chocolates. Developmental toys are also good for the premmie cribs. We decided we would have a huge party when our surviving twin came home from hospital.'

Many parents can feel haunted by the vision of their dead child in the living twin, especially with identical twins. Partners may be especially affected. Right from the start they are usually very involved with twins and most partners are extremely proud of having twins.

Whether the loss is during pregnancy or around the time of birth, don't deny your baby's existence.

- Name your baby.
- Hold and see your baby.
- Talk about your baby.
- Put both babies in the paper, letting people know that your baby who died will also be remembered.
- Take photos of your baby who died – with, and without, their twin and with you. The photos will become very precious in the future.
- Write a letter to your baby expressing your love and your grief and place it in the coffin or in a special book of letters for them. You might continue to write at special moments until you feel you don't need to anymore.
- Have a memorial service or funeral for your baby where you include other children.
- You may need to explain to people that you want to talk about and will be remembering your baby and the twinship – that you don't want them to avoid the subject. Most parents prefer people to say something clumsy rather than nothing at all.

Many families feel the nurses and others who were concerned with the mother's care are the only people who 'knew' their babies, so the mothers often wish to keep in touch and to talk over their loss with them. Mothers often want to talk about the baby, while partners can withdraw and may need encouragement to talk about what has happened. Many mothers report a feeling of loneliness. Having the partner 'room in' in hospital can help. A visit from another mother who has experienced the loss of a baby can also be helpful. Psychologist Michael Carr-Gregg wrote,'This is one of those situations in which our society does not recognise the significance of loss and allow somebody to grieve properly; and for men who have suffered the loss of a newborn their grief is particularly disenfranchised.'

Make use of:

- the hospital chaplain
- the bereavement counsellors in the hospital
- your other children may also benefit from counselling and being given the opportunity to grieve
- your family and friends around you at this time can also help – just being there can be a great comfort and support
- your doctors – ask them questions
- support groups and others who have lost babies and also felt that same intense hurt – specifically SANDS or Bonnie Babes (see Resources, pages 340–47)
- AMBA or NZMBA bereavement contact
- books on coping with grief and helping children to cope with grief

Grieving takes a lot of energy. Give yourself time and say yes to help. Bereaved parents also need time alone together to cry, talk and comfort each other.

When a child loses a twin

Twins can spend almost all, if not all, their time together. They usually see more of each other than they do of either of their parents or of anyone else. If one twin dies, the effect on the surviving twin can be devastating. If the two children have had no experience of being separated, this loss will be even greater. A child whose twin died in the perinatal period may later feel distress, anxiety or curiosity. If their parents cannot talk about it, they should generally seek out someone who can. All surviving twins should hear about their twinship, preferably from the start. They may ask questions, feel angry with their twin for deserting them, angry for causing unhappiness in the family, angry for making them feel guilty. Maybe even anger towards the parents for 'allowing' them to die.

Many grieving parents find the survivor's disturbed behaviour extremely stressful. The surviving twin needs close attention and careful reassurance. Some children believe they are in some way responsible for the death of their twin. A surviving twin may feel guilty that he or she was the one chosen to live. After the bereavement, their choice may seem to be either to exist painfully as half a person or to experience 'survivor guilt' and strive to make up to their parents for the loss, trying to live for two, and setting unrealistic goals leading to inevitable failure.

Some mothers overprotect the survivor, some reject him or her, others do both. Parents often disagree on how to handle the surviving twin. Joining the local twins club for contacts can be helpful.

If one twin is ill, the healthy twin can be involved in the illness and death. She or he will grasp what her level of development will allow. Generally, children under three sense something is wrong but don't really understand what it is. Three to six-year-olds understand someone has gone but think they can return. Six to nine-year-olds understand death but some think the dead person may still return. Nine to twelve-year-olds understand the idea and the permanence of death.

Parents have to decide whether children should attend the funeral or see the dead sibling. Sometimes children are encouraged to become very involved in making or choosing things to put in the coffin. It can be reassuring for some children to see their sibling looking peaceful after they have died.

ANOTHER MUM SAYS 'At first after our son died, his twin brother would be psychotic about going to the cemetery. He understood that his brother was there. It took years for him to let us talk about him. If we talked about when they were young he'd say, 'There's only one, there's only me.' They were so different but after his brother died, our son took on some of his expressions.'

A TWIN SAYS 'Of course at the time I don't even remember the funeral. There was one but I was kept at home. I wish I'd been allowed to go. Even if I couldn't remember a thing about it, just knowing I was actually there would make me feel better now. I feel I've been permanently denied any feelings for my sister. I believe for the sake of memories, and because they are members of the family, children should be taken to funerals regardless of their age.'

Remembering the twin who died

ANOTHER MUM SAYS 'We don't know how to tell our son about his twin brother. I'd like to know that he knows. My mum died around the same time and she was also a really big part of our family. We talk about how we carry them around in our hearts, so they're with us all the time. I wear a necklace every day with a charm for each of my babies. We also buy something for our lost baby to go on the Christmas tree each year and a book for the family on his birthday.'

Older siblings and the loss of a twin

Telling all the world you are going to be the older brother or sister of twins is really special. When one or more dies, especially at birth, the impact on the older child can include feelings like:

- You've lost your mum who is still in hospital.
- You've lost your dad who is so occupied with grief and arranging the funeral.
- You've lost that specialness everyone has been speaking about for months.
- You're not important anymore because Mum and Dad are grieving and not focussing on you or explaining things to you.

The death of a twin in later childhood where the older child is more conscious of the parents' intense grief may mean he'll strive to conceal his own emotions so as not to add to the burden. Support and bereavement counselling from the outset can help avoid difficulties for other children and ease family tensions.

ANOTHER MUM SAYS 'Up until age 14, when their older brother met anyone, within the first couple of sentences he'd say, 'I used to have twin brothers, now there's only one.' In discussions at school he was always very open about his brother, who died at three years and seven months. He had just started school when his brother died. It was a very difficult year for him. His prep teacher was wonderful. He used to take his puppet to sit on the seat next to him at school. Six months later his teacher was so excited because he smiled.'

Which one is which?

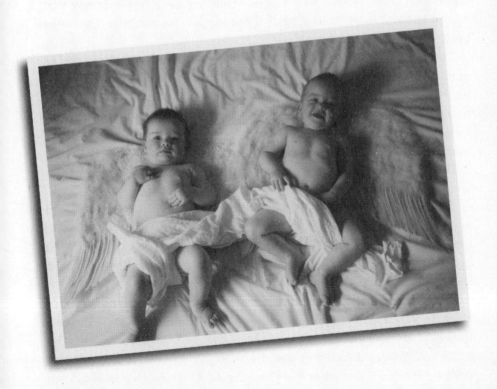

THE TWIN SITUATION

THE TWIN SITUATION: OUR STORIES

As individuals we think we know who we are. We see ourselves as unique and think we choose who we are. Twins raise questions about what forms our own identity.

We find ourselves staring at twins. We want to know about their relationship. Perhaps their lack of obvious differences suggests we may not have much influence on our individuality.

Katrina: I found that many people dismissed my concerns about having two babies at once with comments like 'My two are 12 months apart which is the same as having twins.' For a long time I wondered if having twins is any different from having two children. I was relieved to hear other parents of twins, who've also had two children close together, say that having twins is much harder, 'four times harder' for one and 'ten times harder' according to another.

To get my girls out of the car and into the childcare centre, I needed to get each of them out of their car seats, put each of them in the pram, battle through the doors, then leave the pram and walk one down the corridor and into the nursery and run back to fetch the other. This wasn't a smooth start to their childcare day and often resulted in both being in tears because I had to leave each of them at some point. Taking the pram back to the car I'd see other mothers strolling in with a baby on their hip. Everything I did seemed to be harder.

I've enjoyed all the attention we attract, we are often stopped and admired. Most people have a twin story they want to share. When we first moved to the city, I could wheel the babies to the local shops and talk to people all day. When we took the girls out in separate strollers we received no special attention, it was quite disconcerting.

I have pangs of sadness when I feel my girls might be missing out because they are twins: that they have had to wait, take turns and share their mummy and that people can't tell them apart. All the kids at crèche could say 'Ella' but couldn't get their tongue around 'Charlotte' who became known as the 'other Ella'. I wondered if I'd made a mistake in not giving them both easy names.

When the girls became more mobile they would come to me for cuddles. Ella would always be the first for a big hug. Charlotte would turn away and whinge. At first I was heartbroken and worried that she didn't want physical contact. I started to let Ella wait and to cuddle Charlotte first. I saw an immediate turnaround in Charlotte. Since then she has been wildly affectionate. Her first word was 'Ella'!

I will never understand the extent of the impact they have on each other, but I am confident that they will be happy being twins. They will always be close and already look after each other. They have a genuine affection for each other and I watch their relationship grow while their individuality develops.

Despite the parenting challenges, I'm now thrilled I have twins. As they have grown older life is becoming more balanced. Our children are a huge source of pride and wonder, now I feel it's a lot more interesting than one-at-a-time! My husband has had to be much more involved than many new dads. He puts his family first. When he comes home from work, two delighted little girls run to greet 'Daddy'.

Louise: I was so happy to be pregnant after IVF treatment and news of twins felt like drawing the lucky straw. I was having twins, two babies, I definitely wanted them both. I never compared myself to those having one baby. In the early days it wasn't the girls but 'the situation' that was difficult – when they cried together, were sick at the same time or wouldn't sleep at the same time. Learning the ropes on two at once is very hard work. I felt there was no time to relax and 'enjoy' them. I was too busy to just lie on the floor with them.

It's always been natural to see them as completely separate. They look different, have different interests and have always had different temperaments. They're so often physically close, sharing a chair to watch TV, hopping into bed together. I wonder if this has an influence on how comfortable they'll be with themselves physically as they grow up.

The other twin quality I hope for is an ability to collide with someone then recover immediately – after a big squabble, they're straight back to being friends. Maybe they'll have a healthy approach to an argument being just an argument and be quick with forgiveness and understanding.

When I introduce my girls to people I introduce one, then wait for the hello and name exchanges before introducing the second. It's a small but important way to encourage differentiation. We regularly take them out separately, usually only to the milk bar or to do those little things where getting two into, out of, into and out of the car seems more than the situation warrants. They love being alone with Mum or alone with Dad. 'I'm so happy, Mummy' or 'I love you, Daddy' is said spontaneously at these times. They understand it's turn-taking and they always know whose turn it is.

The girls receive matching outfits as gifts and somehow they always work out between themselves who owns what. One owns both pairs of embroidered denim jeans while the other owns both pink floral tops. They never dress the same and I doubt that it will ever occur to them to dress the same.

I have two girls who are so different from each other and expect to be different from each other. Sometimes they'll choose the same colour ice-cream but it's because they both want it. I don't feel any pressure to treat them the same, love them in the same way, give them the same things. I want to give both of them everything they want and need and so far they both want and need very different things.

When I meet adult twins, my first question is, 'Do you get on well?' or 'Are you close?' I'm hoping they'll be the best of friends.

The clichés

The myths about twins can be very frustrating for parents. People can assume all sorts of things about you and your twins that are quite at odds with reality. One popular book on raising toddlers suggests that twins are easier than two singletons who are a year or two apart because twins often share a room, so are not as likely to have sleep problems. We hear comments in the street, passers-by can't help but offer their opinions.

Twins ... I wish I'd had twins, twice as nice, god blesses twins on those who can cope, twins must be so much better – you get it all over and done with quickly, double trouble, you've got your hands full, how do you manage? better you than me, at least you don't know any better, which one is more dominant? who is the oldest? two peas in a pod ...

What is so different about parenting twins?

The additional concerns parents of twins face before their babies are even born, are a higher-risk pregnancy and a greater likelihood of pre-term birth. The added cost of two in nappies at once, two bassinettes, cots, high chairs, car seats is different and can also be stressful. Parents who have other children are often more concerned about the impact on siblings.

Once the babies arrive, the frustrations of looking after them can include the amount of time spent on day-to-day tasks, and the seemingly impossible task of settling two upset babies. Lack of sleep can be multiplied – some say not twice as tired but two squared, so four times as tired.

During the toddler years, two children who are at the same stage of development can mean two toddlers wanting to be carried, two very messy eaters, double the toilet-training accidents, two toddlers resisting getting into the car, two tantrums at once, two toddlers darting on to the road and two toddlers wanting to slowly and carefully put on their own shoes. They can also give each other ideas and egg each other on.

Later, praising one child without hurting the feelings of the other and managing different levels of achievement can present difficulties for parents and of course there's the enormous decision of whether to keep them in the same class at school.

The tendency to compare twins causes some parents to worry unnecessarily when both their children are within the normal range. Far too often twins are compared with each other rather than with their peers. Finding the balance between meeting the separate needs of two individuals, without squandering their twinship is often a concern for parents of twins.

ANOTHER MUM SAYS 'People don't understand how hard it is, they just think it's cute.'

ANOTHER DAD SAYS 'If I'm home early I sit on the floor and play with who ever wants me. Both either want you or don't want you at once, it's never one at a time. If one crawls up to me, the other has to climb onto me. They both want to be in my face. It's when you're stretched emotionally and physically that the magnitude of having two babies really hits you.'

ANOTHER MUM SAYS 'And now the pay off of twinship is coming through. We have done the hardest yards first – and survived – and we're now coasting very nicely. The girls are so much easier to manage now for the same reason they were so much hard yakka at the start – they're each at the same stage. And as the chore list has dropped away (no more bottle-washing, food-mashing, nappy-changing etc.) my time has become freer to actually do things with them, explore their individual personalities and just enjoy them.'

So, is having twins any different from having two children close in age? Twins are usually reaching the same milestones at around the same time as each other. These milestones are often later than in singleton babies. With two singletons, the elder is usually walking before the younger is mobile. Likewise, the elder is likely to be sleeping through the night before the new baby arrives. Two children may be in nappies and very needy of parental attention, but the elder can also sit and play with some toys or watch a video for a little while, providing some parental respite. Managing two newborns, two babies then two toddlers at once is demanding.

A twin shares the resources that are usually given to one child at that particular age of development. So much has to be shared. They usually learn very quickly to accept sharing and to take turns in the triangle.

ANOTHER MUM SAYS   'In some ways it's like having two children but twins get ideas from each other and encourage each other. One wouldn't think of undressing herself without the other's input. They gang up together and they constantly bicker. Even if there are two toys exactly the same, one of them will want both.'

ANOTHER MUM SAYS   'My friends with singleton babies don't talk to me about their babies as much because I've had twins. I think they feel as though they must have it easier and shouldn't grumble to me about what's troubling them. Perhaps they feel as though I'll turn on them and say, 'You think YOU'VE got problems'. I don't feel that way at all. We all have our challenges. Twins means your life changes more radically faster. By the same token you can regain a sense of equilibrium faster once they grow more independent. I never wanted to be at home for ten years while I had a family and I got what I wished for. Although I didn't expect the gap to be 30 minutes!'

Managing your twins' behaviour

Behaviour can be a much bigger issue for parents of twins. Twins may not want as much positive feedback from their parents when they get it from each other. Rather than trying to please their parents, they can please each other by doing things that may not please their parents, perhaps behaving in inappropriate ways. Parents of twins often need to use more obvious verbal instructions and physical separation to encourage particular behaviour. You may like to speak with them differently and separately, rather than the same and together.

ANOTHER MUM SAYS   'Sometimes I feel there are more arguments for me to resolve, because they're twins. They get jealous of each other and fight over toys or me. It can be so exhausting when I've just gone through the process of disciplining one, even if it's just a rebuke for touching something they shouldn't, because the other always has to 'touch it too' and I have to go through it all again.'

Professor David Hay says, 'Don't encourage behaviour from one twin designed to get attention away from the other. While few parents would do this consciously, every time you respond to this approach you are encouraging its recurrence in both twins. Twins need to learn two things more than other children, namely to wait and to take turns.' He gives the example of two-year-old twins in country Victoria who seemed to be suffering from an incredible neurological syndrome where they were always falling down. For several days they were dropping like flies. There wasn't anything wrong with them – they were enjoying the attention.

> **REMEMBER**
>
> 'The main problem for twins is that there are two of them.'
> Professor David Hay

Treating your twins as individuals

'No matter how identical the children are life cannot provide exactly the same for each child. Multiples have differing needs at different times and it is therefore unfair to try and treat them in the same way.'
Pat Preedy, in *Twin and Triplet Psychology*

'No matter how tantalisingly alike we may be, no one crosses the boundary between being alike and being the same.'
Lawrence Wright, *Twins*

Parents of twins can be concerned about what is fair and whether they should be treated equally. Does that mean they should be treated the same? Parents of twins can feel the pressure to reward both twins, even when only one has achieved. Or they can withhold the reward from one twin in order to save the feelings of the other. Twins may need additional support from you to cope with the feelings associated with the times when life for them simply is not fair. At the same time, as they are expected to be the same, they are looked at closely for differences. They are constantly being compared with each other. At every stage of development a comparison is made. Who was born first? Who's rolling first? Standing first? Walking first? Which one is faster or slower, taller or smaller, bossier or quieter? Which one is dominant? Who was born first? Which one is bigger?

Everyone asks. Does this mean the comparisons are important? Are they using the answers to draw conclusions? Measuring something? Why do they want to know? Like most siblings, twins can often compete for attention by differentiating themselves. Where twins appear to be opposites, they may have chosen polarisation as a means of establishing their own identities. This can create the danger that they may be labelled the 'good' and 'bad' twin.

If twins are treated as two separate individuals and encouraged to have their own friends and activities, as well as shared ones, this can help them to develop the skills they need when their twin is not available.

TO HELP YOUR TWINS TO DEVELOP AS INDIVIDUALS

- Make individual eye-contact with each child when you're speaking with them.
- Address the children individually rather than as a pair.
- Present the children to others as individuals rather than as one unit.
- Speak to them as individuals and encourage them to respond in complex sentences.
- Reward them for their individual achievements.
- Compare their development with their peer group and not with each other.
- Help them to develop their own friends and interests, arranging opportunities for them to play with their peers without their twin.
- Arrange for them to have time away from their twin with separate outings and experiences.
- Talk about the good things about being twins and celebrate joint as well as individual achievements.

ANOTHER MUM SAYS 'It's easy with my two older children to treat them differently but with the twins I have to resist the urge to treat them the same. I always have to take a deep breath and think about how individual they are, their different abilities and temperaments.'

A TWIN SAYS 'We were always fierce rivals as well as the best of friends.'

ANOTHER MUM SAYS 'I love them both the same but for different reasons. I think part of the twin thing is needing to identify their differences. I look at them and wonder why it was they were born together. I think one is all heart and the other is the light that radiates from the heart. One can't exist without the other. I'm very keen for them to be seen as individuals. It helps that they look so different. But I also want to embrace the fact that they're twins and forever interconnected.'

ANOTHER MUM SAYS 'My boys don't even look like brothers, and have been described as Merv Hughes and Michael Leunig. Most people don't believe they are twins. They have developed at different rates, they are now a year apart at school, they've always had separate friends, but their relationship is really close. The way they interact with each other, you can tell they are twins.'

Twins' friendships

'The twin relationship is unique and complex according to situation and activity, all their friendships will be affected by the fact that they are a twin.'

Pat Preedy, in *Twin and Triplet Psychology*

When twins are younger they mostly share the same friends, but pairs can often stick together to the exclusion of others. It's important for your children's self-esteem that they form relationships with children other than their twin. If one twin develops a particular friendship, this may lead to jealousy and a feeling of great loss in the other. In developing their relationships as individuals and as twins, they learn to understand that sometimes each will have different experiences. When inviting friends over for play, many parents invite two friends rather than one, to help even the field. Not only is it good for you to know other parents of twins, but it's also helpful for your twins to know other twins. They often receive a lot of attention for being twins. It helps them to know they're not the only ones, there are others like them who come in pairs.

Birthdays

Birthdays present a dilemma for parents of twins. Not just the twins' own birthday, but also their friends' birthday parties. Talk to your friends and family about recognising the twins as two individuals at birthday time.

You could consider:

- A birthday cake each, even if it's a cup cake with their own candle each.
- Separate presents. Some will be to share, like a table and chairs or a video, but each child could have their own present to open.
- A birthday card each.
- Singing Happy Birthday to each separately.
- When one twin is invited to a party, but not the other, take one to the party and the other out with you on a special adventure.
- When both twins are invited to a party, let each of them buy a present for the birthday child.

Spending time apart

Many parents help their twins to establish their own identity and a sense of independence by providing opportunities for them to spend time apart. It's also excellent for their language development, social skills and their sense of identity. Taking them out alternately on their own means they feel safe spending time apart. The earlier you start, the more easily they'll adapt to spending time without their twin. It doesn't have to be a big deal or expensive excursion, it can become part of the weekly routine.

Preschool and kindergarten

Starting preschool or kindergarten can be a major change in the lives of parents and children. It can be the first time children have extensive contact with children other than their siblings, and also the first time others encounter twins. The preschool or kindergarten experience will help you decide whether your children are ready for school and help identify any potential problems in their development before they start school.

Preschool offers many opportunities for individual and separate experiences for the two children. They can form relationships with other children in a group setting and there are many opportunities for language to develop.

When choosing a kindergarten or preschool, talk with the teachers about their experiences in caring for twins. Tell them how you prefer your twins to be managed. Help carers and other children to distinguish identical twins by giving them name tags, colour coding them or providing some other way to tell them apart. Research shows that just knowing they are twins affects people's memory, so that identifying them as individuals and calling them by their names can seem difficult.

Are your twins ready for school?

Children need lots of stimulation and social interaction to help them become more ready for school. Mixing with other children, swimming lessons, visiting the zoo all broaden their horizons and help to prepare them. If you're unsure whether one or both are ready for school, it's better to repeat a year of kindergarten and delay beginning school.

Before children start school they need:
- Verbal skills – parents can read with their children, emphasising how much fun and how important reading is.
- Some physical skills and independence – can they tie their own shoes, can they take responsibility for their belongings?
- An ability to wait and take turns – parents can teach them not to distract each other, let one finish a puzzle without the other messing it up.
- Some independence – parents can give them some time apart.

Some parents of twins delay the children's start to school, particularly if they were pre-term babies. If one is ready, but the other is not, it's generally considered better to hold them both back. Holding one back and not the other can have disastrous implications. If they've started school and it's obvious early in the first term that they are not ready, you can take them out during the first term. Some local councils have field officers who can help assess your child for their readiness for school. Or you can discuss it with other professionals including a maternal child health nurse, kindergarten teacher or child carers.

When planning your twins' education, consider:
- prematurity, their preschool development or health problems
- their previous experiences of separation and the reaction of each child
- their relationships with other children
- competitiveness – are they always striving to beat each other
- whether they have a significant difference in ability or whether one child opts out
- whether the twins are polarised and choose to go to opposite extremes – quiet/noisy, outgoing/shy
- whether one restricts the other
- their dominance/dependence

The 'Twins in School' website (www.twinsandmultiples.org) launched in 2001 is a collaboration between Australian psychologist Professor David Hay, who has worked with multiple birth families for 27 years, and Dr Pat Preedy, a leading school principal in the UK. The site provides a wealth of information about helping twins develop as individuals and preparing them for school. It is useful for parents and teachers.

Preparing the teacher and the school

It can be helpful to tell the teacher a bit about each child, to help her/him get to know them better. Teachers may need to be encouraged to regard your twins as individuals and to refer to them by name. Explain that you'd like the teacher to evaluate the progress of each child in the context of their peers, rather than comparing them to each other. At parent-teacher interview times, schedule separate meetings for each twin, even if it's the first five minutes about one, then the second about the other. By avoiding twin comparisons when speaking with teachers, you may discourage the teachers from comparing them. Avoid saying, 'She is the quieter one . . .'

Separate or keep together?

Each year over 7000 twin children start school in Australia and their parents face the dilemma of whether or not to separate them. A 'Twins in School' project was undertaken to establish the first reliable evidence about separation of twins in primary schools. The main message from the survey was that the best policy is no policy. What works well for one family may be totally inappropriate for the next. Decisions about separation of twins in school are best made a year at a time, based on what is best for that family.

Unless there is a reason to separate them, keeping twins together at the start of school is the current recommended practice. Many parents will buddy up their single children with a friend for the start of school. Twinship just means the children have a ready-made pal to ease their transition. You may choose to keep them together the first year and then reassess the situation. While you want them to be individuals, you don't want to destroy their twin bond. Remember that school is only a part of life. Developing as an individual does not depend solely upon separation from your twin at school. The attitudes of parents and teachers are much more important. It's up to us to set the standards for our twins – it's how we react and value each child that will impact on them.

Some parents express a preference for their twins to be separated but may not be prepared for the possibility of an adverse reaction from the children. Separation often allows the dependent child to blossom while the dominant one can fret for a time at having lost their major role. The children need to be prepared for separation with some time apart prior to school and separate visits to prepare for school.

It is advisable to separate twins if:

- one twin is dominant to the degree that the other is almost dependent
- they greatly restrict each other's activities
- they are prone to combining to form a powerful unit causing disruption

ANOTHER MUM SAYS 'After hearing our girls being called the wrong name for the first five years of their lives the decision to separate them at school was quite easy. We thought it was high time they had a chance to become the individuals that they are. The chance to form their own friendships, have their own teachers and the excitement of coming home with their own stories of the day at school was an opportunity we all looked forward to.'

ANOTHER MUM SAYS   'I decided to separate our children so they could develop their own personalities and make their own friends. Being boy/girl twins I felt this was very important. It turned out to be the right choice for us and again in Grade One they have continued in separate classes. They still play together at times and can tell me a lot about each other's day but they work at their own pace and love to have their own classrooms to show me.'

Language development

Language development in twins is often different from, rather than inferior to, that of single children. Twins are usually talking with two others rather than one so can be very good at social conversation and at using personal pronouns. Most twins have no problems in learning to talk and many twins are ahead of singles in their speech, but it is sensible to keep an eye on the language progress of twins as, statistically, they are more likely to have problems than single-born children.

Twins can have less one-on-one time with adults who are busy with two or more children. They are so familiar with each other that they can use ways other than speech to communicate and can reinforce each other's incorrect pronunciation or grammar. Twins can also speak loudly and simply in order to get their parents' attention, and often interrupt each other's conversation.

If there are delays in their language development, it is often in their ability to articulate their thoughts and feelings correctly. Their sentences can be shorter and baby talk can persist for longer.

Language delays can have an impact on whether twins are ready to start school and can affect their achievement at school and their reading ability.

Many factors can affect how children learn to talk, including hearing impairment, long periods of illness, lack of stimulation or, as can happen with twins, one sibling who talks for both. It's important to investigate with a speech therapist the cause of any language delay, and the earlier the better.

TIPS TO HELP DEVELOP CHILDREN'S SPEECH

- Ask questions of, and actively listen to, each child – make eye contact and speak to each, not two at a time.
- Encourage each to speak for his or herself – if one asks for a banana, don't automatically give one to the other.
- Pay attention when your children talk to you. Listen and respond, making it a pleasant interaction for them.
- Talk all the time. Repeat the names of objects you see. Talk while you play. Explain what you're doing, where you're going and why.
- Ask daycare workers or extended family to speak one-on-one with your children.
- Have one-on-one time, particularly reading. If you've only got the two kids and there are two parents, it's a good habit for you to go to separate places and read to one each every night.
- If you suspect a problem, early intervention by a speech therapist may help dramatically.

Speech therapy can make a difference

If pursuing treatment with a speech therapist, ask what experience they have with twins. There are particular issues, for example, if only one child is getting therapy, she may be upset at being singled out or her twin may be upset at missing out. All the work by the therapist and the parents may be in vain if the interactions between the twins continue in their old and incorrect speech.

ANOTHER MUM SAYS　'At two, I was concerned that their speech was just mumble-jumble and few words made sense. I had an older child who talked all the time – and I talked all the time – so I assumed we wouldn't have any problems. But at two, it was obvious they had major problems. I could understand other two-year-olds, but I could hardly understand a word mine said. One didn't make sense and the other said very little. I was particularly concerned about my son not speaking much and he didn't interact with people much either. The speech therapist assessed them as being six months behind. In some ways I was relieved when the problem was diagnosed as it confirmed what I had been telling people, but I was also upset by it. I remember sitting down on the steps at home and crying. Although I knew we could fix the problem, part of me had been hoping the speech therapist would have told me that nothing was wrong. The therapist was unable to give a reason for why their speech was delayed other than that they were twins. I wanted to know what had caused it. Did I talk to them, read to them, sing to them enough? Should I have taken them out more? The speech therapist said they didn't know what caused it, it was a twin thing, but that with therapy they could bring them up to scratch by the time they started school. They started half-hour sessions of speech therapy once a fortnight. A lot of the therapy involved working with me and telling all the family what we needed to do to help the twins to develop language skills.

There were two main things. Firstly, stop anticipating their needs all the time and get them to ask for things they wanted. I needed to give them more choices so they were forced to ask for what they wanted. For example, I always selected their clothes for them because they weren't really interested in choosing what they wanted to wear. But I had to offer them choices and ask them questions to get them to speak. Secondly, all the family and anyone who cared for the children needed to talk constantly – even if it was not to the twins but just around them. The idea was not to try to force them to speak but to let them just pick up what was being said around them. I remember I would be going to the supermarket in the car and I would be saying, 'We are going to do the shopping at the supermarket, and look at that house over there.' Then one day when we were going in the car one of them said 'shopping' and I nearly drove off the road in shock. The speech therapist also recommended that the twins attend creche for a day or two a week so they could learn to co-operate with other children and talk to them. After six months of therapy, the twins moved into a language group with six other children with speech delays and they did group activities which they really enjoyed. They have since moved into a dance and movement group which is an extension of the language group and is made up of children with delays in other areas including other premmies. Their speech is now going well – they talk non-stop.'

Going into hospital

If one twin is admitted to hospital, it may be easier on the whole family for both to be admitted. If illness in hospital is the first experience of separation for twins, it can be an extremely painful experience and can amplify the sense of crisis. The healthy twin should be closely involved with his brother's or sister's illness and, where appropriate, be reassured that he or she will not catch the same illness or die. A toddler separated from her twin by a hospital visit reacts in a similar way to a child separated from her mother. She cuts herself off from emotion and rejects the person who she feels has rejected her. Visits by the twin will help reassure her, even if she reacts badly to them. On her return there could be anger directed towards her twin as well as towards the parent.

ANOTHER MUM SAYS   'Just before our son's second birthday he was admitted to hospital with septic arthritis in his left knee. He was in hospital for a little under three weeks, with a couple of days home in the middle. One of us had to be with him 24 hours a day and fortunately my husband's employers were very supportive. He took the first week off and we tagged to and from the hospital. My mother-in-law came from interstate to stay with the other one, which was a great help. Toward the end of his stay we were more organised and I did the day shift and my husband did the night shift. He would come home, shower and go off to work. After work he would spend some time with our other son until he went to bed and would then come in to the hospital and I would go home for the night. It was a difficult time for all of us. It is hard to say what impact it had on the boys, but during the first week our other son would sleep in his brother's cot every night. I think that if they were separated like that now (four months later) the effect on them would be more apparent as they interact with each other a lot more now.'

What is it about being a twin that makes it different?

Twins spend almost all of their time together and from conception they share everything. This is a unique psychological experience. They have a relationship which they often identify as very positive but it is also very complex and can include ambivalent feelings.

A TWIN SAYS 'Competition can be good but it can also be exhausting. You are always trying to prove you are the smarter, thinner, brighter one, not the fatter, dumber, duller one. Parents of twins should treat them like brothers and sisters and not encourage too much comparison.'

A TWIN SAYS 'As a twin you have double the wardrobe.'

A TWIN SAYS 'I don't know what it would be like not to be a twin, being a twin is all I know I don't have to search out friendships with that close bond. I have it ready made.'

A TWIN SAYS 'At school everyone compared us so we overcompensated by trying to be really different from each other, we denied our own personalities. When we reached our thirties we felt more comfortable.'

A TWIN SAYS 'She never says what she's thinking but I know what she's thinking.'

A TWIN SAYS 'As teenagers our twinship was more negative. I was rebellious and she was straight-laced. I used to think she was very down on me. We had different friends at school and went to separate secondary schools for the last two years. The competition between us was overt but in many ways caused us both to work harder at everything. There was definitely some jealousy. We speak to each other a few times a week and about ten times on our birthday. My birthday is not just about me it's about both of us.'

A TWIN SAYS 'I get emotional even thinking about it, but I can't imagine what it must be like to lose a twin. It makes me sick thinking about it. It would feel like part of me had died. Nothing would ever be the same.'

A TWIN SAYS   'Being an identical twin was special. We were always stared at in the street and got loads of attention – when we were little it was fun. Then when we grew up, people would come up to us separately thinking we were the other one. You get used to it, and have some bizarre experiences. We now live in different countries, but he's still more than a brother. He's a soulmate, really.'

Twins grow up. The challenges for parents of twins become much less physical and relentless while the difficulties associated with being a twin change and remain. As children become adults, they no longer depend on their parents, ideally replacing this dependence with a mature and equal relationship. Twins also alter their relationship with their parents but also have the added emotional journey of separating from their co-twin. Parents of twins can make this transition easier by gently providing opportunities to encourage a sense of autonomy and independence at an early age, while respecting the twinship bond. The happiest twins may be those who manage to continue sharing a bond and having a lifelong friendship while allowing each other the physical and emotional freedom to develop this autonomy.

Actually, there are three . . .

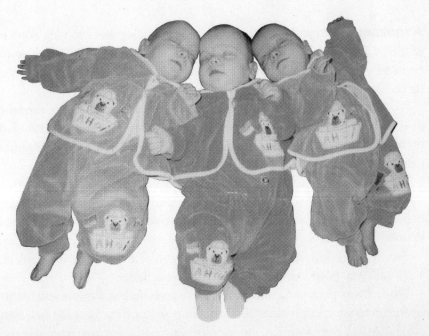

TRIPLETS

Triplets: Families' Stories

At an AMBA national convention a number of parents of triplets asked us to include them in the next edition of *Twins*. Many parents of triplets were willing to share their stories, hoping that other families would find their experiences encouraging.

Triplet facts

YEAR	TRIPLETS AND HIGHER ORDER MULTIPLES BORN IN AUSTRALIA
1982	33
1987	65
1992	112
1997	107
2002	83*

* This equals one in 2973 births
Source: Australian Bureau of Statistics

A mother's story: 'It was a shock finding out we were having triplets at the 13-week scan. The doctor thought I might be having twins because of the results from the blood test, but I never contemplated three.

My babies had all just waved to me during a scan on the screen then the doctors offered me a selective reduction asking if I wanted to abort two of them. I felt it was all or nothing. If I could turn back time I wouldn't change the decision but I would never want to have triplets again.

I felt remarkably calm after learning about the three babies. I started thinking about how to organise the house and the car. My husband was panicking and felt we should consider selective reduction. He felt scared that they'd be disabled. We didn't talk on the way home from the hospital.

People don't know what to say when you're pregnant with triplets. They say 'you poor thing' but I thought I was lucky.

While I was pregnant, simple tasks like pushing the supermarket trolley began to seem impossible, I'd be huffing and puffing after the first two aisles, my feet were swollen, my tummy big. I got heartburn mopping the floor. I couldn't turn in bed or sleep. I was told I'd be bedridden after 20 weeks but that didn't happen. At 30 weeks I'd had enough, so I called the hospital and went in for a rest. I saw struggling babies in the intensive care nursery but I'd done all I could possibly do. I felt like there was nothing left in my body for the babies. At 32 weeks one of my babies got distressed and I needed an emergency caesarean. I'll always have a soft spot for my little boy who got stressed and helped bring on their birth.

The operating suite was like a stadium. Three people per baby, plus doctors, assistants, anaesthetist – they all came to the table and politely introduced themselves. My obstetrician walked in with gum boots above her knees and a type of raincoat and long gloves—she looked like a butcher. She had to climb some steps to get up to my belly. I didn't recognise my husband when he walked in with his robe and mask. The doctor held up each baby for a quick glance then they were straight to their cribs for medical attention.

They were skinny little babies needing to be gavage fed and in isolettes. They got constant pin-pricks in their heels, it broke my heart. I felt guilty seeing them thinking I should have kept them in my belly longer. Two days after the birth a pregnant mother in hospital asked me, 'When's yours due?' I was no longer pregnant but my stomach was still bigger than hers. I felt insulted because I thought I was skinny!

The babies were in hospital for five weeks. I went home after five days because of my toddler. The hospital was congested and they said they were moving my babies to another hospital. They had to get my consent and I wouldn't give it. I didn't want new staff looking after my boys and a new hospital exposing them to risk of infections. The hospital staff said I'd have to take one of them home but I didn't want to separate them. He was ready but the other two weren't ready to be discharged as they weren't feeding properly. I was assertive and said, 'You can't make me take my baby'. I knew we wouldn't manage with two children at home and two in hospital. I was protecting my children and the alternative would have created too much panic and chaos.

The car was a big issue. With our toddler and the triplets, we needed to accommodate four baby car seats and two twin prams. We fitted out a commercial van with enough seats and extra anchor points so there was still room for shopping in the back.

Having a baby already made me decide not to breastfeed the triplets but I made the decision to express for one month so they would get the colostrum. I expressed at home and my husband would take it into hospital in the morning. I'd go in later to bathe and dress them.

The hospital staff were more panicky than me about going home with the babies. I felt confident I'd be fine. The midwives came to us for home visits and provided the hospital's disposable nappies for a few months.

I didn't want to be dependent on other people to be able to look after my children. I didn't have family help and the hospital social worker organised the council to provide home help which meant a cleaner for three hours once a fortnight.

My parenting style changed completely between the first baby and the next three. I rocked my first to sleep. None of the triplets ever fell asleep in my arms – as soon as they were fed and had a nappy change they were back to bed. I'd pat their bottoms a couple of times, make no eye contact and then shut the door behind me – you can't rock three babies. I did a lot more limit setting. We took our first baby everywhere, but when you've got three babies, you don't go anywhere – you're too tired and you can't push two twin prams on your own.

I had one four-hour sleep once a day because my husband did the 11 pm feed. After six months of round-the-clock feeding we were exhausted. I was saved by a neighbour who did the night shift once a week. Then a friend contributed a night shift that meant we had two decent nights sleep a week.

My neighbour also set up a roster system with helpers from her church. Every day for months somebody came in to help. They could do things like take my older son for a walk or stay with the babies and bottle feed while I did the shopping. Nobody wanted to feed my littlest one because he took so long, everyone wanted the big boy who was more like a normal sized baby.

I no longer had any privacy. People were folding my undies, opening my drawers, the fridge and my cupboards. I had an instant family invading my space and all these other helpers. There were always too many people. I had no time on my own. The boys were born in February. The first time we all went out as a family was in June – we all walked up to the pharmacy to get some Panadol, then walked back. Even now, Saturdays are really important to me because it's just the kids and me. I've claimed Saturdays mentally as my space and I don't tell anyone – it's the only secret I've got left.

A real estate agent knocked on the door one day and wanted to come in to look at the triplets. I told her to go away as they were babies, not freaks. These days we have an electronic button and intercom system on the front gate. It's maximum security to keep the boys in and intruders out.

It was very important to me to treat them all well. I made sure they all had a hot bath with clean fresh water. Each had their own bowl and spoon. This created more work for me but I was still the same person and these things were important to me. I was also still holding on to my true self, the person I was before the 'invasion'. Following my own methods was a way of retaining my sense of self.

I wanted to look nice, wear nice things, do my hair and have a neat home. You don't feel human when your back's sore, and you're sick because you're run down, your hands are dry and split because of all the washing in between nappy changes – two and a half years of that and you feel like crap. When you're doing three hourly feeds with triplets, that leaves half an hour between rounds to cook, clean, sleep, play with our older child and everything else.

Now they're three I'm just a very busy mum. I have four boys in the bath at once, and while they are having fun I run around and clean up the house then they're dressed and go into the lounge while I clean up the bathroom after them. Sometimes I think I should mop the floor less but it's my choice and a clean house is important to me. I don't feel physically dead just mentally dead because it's always 'Mummy, Mummy, Mummy'. It's hard to please four children plus a husband at once.

I'm known as the 'triplet mum' which really annoys me. I don't like the fuss wherever I go. I get funny looks. People ask me, 'How do you tell them apart?' and, 'How do you do it?' but I just have to. I've been asked so many times 'Are they all yours?'. When they ask me 'Are they natural?' I say they look pretty natural to me. The nicest thing somebody said to me is, 'You've got lovely boys, they're a credit to you.'

I look at people complaining about their one child and I think, 'Give me a break!' I could never feel sorry for people with one baby having a bad day. I've lost my heart that way. I try to stay away from those conversations in fear I might say something I may regret. I don't have time for coffees and stuff about buying cute things at the shops – I've got a list a mile long whizzing around my head at all times.

The furniture, the floors and our walls are all either scratched, dented or stained. You can't watch them all the time and it's just not worth trying to keep everything as it was. I put all my 'nice things' away and when I pulled them out again they just looked old-fashioned. I don't stress about material things anymore – it's people who are important and I'd rather invest the time and energy into my children.

I feel my own sense of achievement in parenting triplets and a toddler. They're normal well balanced human beings and I know I've done a good job.

Their need to be the same is overwhelming. If one is wearing his Spiderman pyjamas, the others insist on wearing theirs too. My older son doesn't care if he's wearing something different. If I wanted to give attention to one I couldn't as they're constantly looking for each other. They are more caring of others and inclusive of each other, no one is ever left out. I try to encourage them to claim something for themselves to reduce fights and so they have something to call their own, even if it's the same cup in a different colour.

If one wants to hold my hand, they all need to hold my hand and I've got them tugging at fingers. My identical pair seem content to share me, but their non-identical brother won't. They all want hugs, kisses, praise – I can't kiss one without ensuring all the others get a kiss too. If I praise one for being a good boy, the others will pipe in with 'But I'm a good boy too, Mummy ...' Driving the car, one will say, 'Look Mummy, there's a circus' and I respond with 'Yes, a circus' and then they each have to take their turn to say the circus and I have to reply to each of them. In the car I often wish I could press a button to bring up the sound proof screen between me and the noise in the back.

Time seems never ending. I feel like it has slipped me by. I wish I had more time and that's why I'm always taking photos so I don't forget this time with the boys.

A FAMILY SAYS   'I'm so over the word 'mummy' – but then it's very appropriate because I feel like the living dead.'
Mother, father, boy 4 ½, triplet boys aged 3 ½ (including an identical twin pair).

A mother's story: We'd tried for 18 months to get pregnant and were contemplating fertility treatment when it just happened. I had a normal scan at 12 weeks but then started getting really ill. At my next scan the technician said there were twins. Then he said there's another one. My husband turned white and had his head in his hands. I was just crying, wondering how I would cope and was already starting to worry about the finances. It was total shock.

I adopted a mindset that I could achieve this. I started getting strong and getting organised. We started accumulating as much furniture as we could. I concentrated on getting through the pregnancy.

Triplets are financially crippling. We needed a new car – Chrysler Voyager seemed to offer good leg room, boot space and seats that could be changed around. Life changes drastically with triplets – car, house, friends, financials, lifestyle – so many parents have to change the work they do.

It would have been harder if we hadn't been through feeding and sleeping with an older child. We already knew the fundamentals and the value of patterns and routine. Those skills proved absolutely vital.

During the pregnancy people were saying to our older son that he'd have to be a big brother and help Mummy and Daddy with the three babies. His behaviour changed dramatically. He regressed, with tantrums and aggressive behaviour. We sat down with him and explained that he didn't have to help if he didn't want to and he'd still get to play with his friends and toys. We could see the relief in his face and he returned to his normal self. As well as keeping an eye on our son, we also have my husband's eldest three to consider. We tried to include them as much as we could throughout the pregnancy.

My doctor advised me to leave my work at the bank at 19 weeks. I got very sick, was short of breath and one of the babies' fluid sacs was leaking. I was told to take it easy and couldn't continue to be on my feet. I focused on keeping well and my husband focused on getting organised for the babies' arrival. He seemed to know how hard it was to carry three babies and encouraged me to take it easy.

I first went into labour at 29 weeks, with contractions starting while I was in the bath. There was a shortage of hospital beds and they were going to transfer me interstate. Fortunately they gave me something that stopped the labour and I only had four days in hospital.

At 32 weeks full contractions started and I was already half dilated when we got to the hospital. We'd planned for a caesar so I was given an epidural and one hour later had three babies.

The staff explained to us what was going on during the birth. It is daunting to see so many people in the room. They were quick to reassure us straight away that the babies were relatively healthy. The babies went to intensive care. I felt like I'd been hit by a truck.

I knew my life was going to be different. I didn't want to go home and cope with it. I'd dealt with the pregnancy and the caesar but didn't think at all about how life would be after they were born. I hadn't mentally prepared myself for leaving hospital and coping with triplets.

Having the triplets taught me that life is about change and that I can cope with the unforeseen. The harder you fight against it the harder it is. My life was always so safe and secure, working with the bank for 20 years

Whenever one of the babies stopped breathing or got an infection it was very stressful. They went through breathing difficulties because they were eight weeks early. It was one step forward, two steps back. You can't prepare yourself for that trauma.

I was in tears every day. Having triplets is the most gut-wretching thing I've been through in my life. For the eight weeks they were in hospital I would worry all night. I'd try to get up to the hospital to do feeds. After they'd been in intensive care for six weeks, they were moved to a closer hospital for two weeks.

While pregnant I'd decided not to breastfeed. I'd had a difficult experience with my first baby and felt the best thing was to bottle feed. I also didn't want the responsibility of being the only person who could feed three babies.

Coming home was a complete shock. The first night we had half an hour of sleep between us. We played tag team so we'd both get some sleep. When they were a little bit older we'd do night feeds in turn. I'd go to bed at 7.30 pm, my husband would do the 10 pm feed which took til 1 am. An hour later he'd start the 2 am feed, be in bed 3.30 am til 8.00 am then off to work. I would do the 6 am feed and the day shift.

Initially we enquired about in-home care with the local council, but they didn't provide it. We tried our near neighbouring council where we had more success, and ended up with in-home help.

I had post natal depression so did the best I could in the circumstances. I felt like a failure as a mum because I wasn't coping. My friends stopped coming because they knew someone was here helping and didn't want to intrude. If I went out I felt guilty because I wasn't the one looking after my children. I ended up having panic attacks if I left the house.

When the babies were small and it was round the clock feeding the home help was great – we couldn't have done it ourselves. Organisation and routine are absolutely vital.

The turning point for me was organising family day care as it brought some normality back to my life. Family day care means I can sometimes have a clean home. It's also been great for the triplets because they get out of the house. I wanted to keep them together and they were less likely to get sick if they weren't in a child care centre. The carer takes them to play groups and the playground as she has a car and pram that can accommodate them all. My youngest daughter now goes there too.

My husband had to leave his job in the city. He started his own home business. I looked at going back to work part-time but it wasn't worth it financially or logistically. Family day care means I can shop for groceries, clean, cook and maybe get to the hairdresser. On the days the children are home the house is trashed and I've just had to learn not to worry about it.

We hardly noticed the impact of our fifth baby. The initial pregnancy was a bombshell. I was on the pill. My husband had been to the clinic for a vasectomy and was advised to wait until the triplets were 12 months old. The hardest thing was telling others we were pregnant. People would say we were crazy and were very quick to be negative. We had to dig deep. Our biggest fear was another multiple birth and my first step was an ultrasound. After our daughter was born I was a total mess, crying all the time. I experienced this period of grief and feeling very sorry for myself then ended up having to focus on moving forward.

There isn't enough time to put into relationships. Some people cope with our new life, some don't. Some can't handle the fact that we need help. A lot of people offered help, but actually getting any was difficult. Everybody is busy with their own lives and your own family comes first. My friends know if they want to see me it's easier to come to my place.

Some people make decisions for us thinking they're helping by not inviting us in the first instance. Our family means there's an extra four or five kids for the birthday party. Some people want to associate themselves with us because of the celebrity factor. People like to think they 'know' the triplets.

People say a multiple birth makes or breaks your marriage. Our relationship had a very strong base and our determination has kept us going. Life is hard, work is hard, marriage is hard. We try to go away once a year for five days without the children. Their aunts come from the country to look after the kids. We value most the opportunity to eat a meal together in peace and to sleep in.

We couldn't always see the light at the end of the tunnel, we just had to believe it was there. We had to dig deep to get through to that point where it's not all damn hard work. We just get through one day at a time and still can't see five years down the track.

A downside to parenting triplets is lack of individual bonding, they lose individuality and too often are treated as three-in-one instead of three individuals. They have a very special bond with each other and always have someone to play with. The notoriety of being a triplet is both a positive and a negative. All their life they will have that something special about them.

Before they were born I wondered how on earth I could parent three children at once, and whether I had the capacity to do it well. If I respond to one of the triplets in a certain manner and the others are present I need to give them all the same message: I love you … I love you … I love you … I love you … I love you … It's a constant challenge to try and maintain equilibrium while treating them as individuals. But it's important not to beat yourself up, it's a situation that tests you all the time and all you can do is your best.

Our life is hectic and it's been hard but we wouldn't have it any other way. We have a big family and love it. We feel incredibly fortunate to have eight of the most beautiful children anyone can hope for and love that they're part of our lives.

A FAMILY SAYS It is an enormously special experience that few people get the opportunity to have. It's a massive responsibility and we feel a great sense of achievement. We've been blessed by this opportunity and responsibility.

Mother, father, 8-year-old boy, 3 ½-year-old fraternal triplets (two boys and a girl), 2-year-old girl. The father also has three older children from his previous marriage who stay over every 3rd weekend.

A mother's story: We have a 23-year-old daughter, a 20-year-old daughter and fraternal triplets aged 17 (two girls and a boy). I'm just chomping at the bit to find myself again – it's taken this long. I had five children under six and you don't realise the toll it takes on you until you reflect. Last year I went away for five days with my mum and I started to realise a life away from the family, I'm rediscovering my own identity. I've always been yearning for it but until now it wasn't realistic. It has been nice to spend some time with Mum again and to be a daughter – to have someone nurture me. Now I'm allowing myself to review and move on.

I was mortified when I found out I was expecting triplets. I'll never forget it. It was a big decision to try for a third baby. I'd had two miscarriages and with this pregnancy I didn't feel quite right and I was so big – I expected that I'd lost the baby. At the 10-week ultrasound I went in half expecting news of another lost pregnancy and the doctor spotted twins – then he said, 'Oh my God, there's a third one!' I started crying, Mum was with me and she was horrified. We were making our way out and the doctor had already told everyone in the waiting room. The prep teacher knew before I even got to pick up my daughter and tell her for myself. It was a huge invasion of my privacy and I felt behind the eight ball already. From thinking I wasn't pregnant to everybody knowing I was expecting triplets was too much. Straight away I'd lost control of the situation.

The babies were born at 38 weeks – I had an elective caesar and had to fight my doctor to get a tubal ligation at the same time. As a nurse, I'd attended two triplet vaginal births where the third was stillborn.

I breastfed my babies for the first five months. I'd breastfed my other two so I knew I could breastfeed the triplets. I'd twin feed two then do the third one both sides, on a rotational basis. I started bottles in the evening after five months. I knew breastfeeding was the best thing for them and I'll always be glad I did it, even though it took more time.

I was always confident about establishing the routine. When they were tiny I'd get up at 5.30 am and bathe the triplets, then feed between 6 am and 7 am. They'd go in their bouncinettes and I'd wake the older two to get them ready for kinder and school. We'd do the school run then home for the morning nap, then back for the kinder pick-up. The three learnt to sleep regardless of where they were – they were lugged upstairs into capsules from cots and if they were tired they'd just go to sleep again.

My work as a midwife is time-management focused. This gave me the essential organisational skills needed to manage the home and family. I was never late for anything and everything was always done. There were always clean clothes and cooked meals. You need to think today about what you're doing tomorrow. Everyday I had 'my time'. Between one and three in the afternoon I just did my needlework. I didn't clean or cook and always had the kids in bed. Then it would all start again.

We had strict bed times and afternoon rest times, even if they didn't want to sleep – these things were not negotiable. Bed time was 7 pm so I could then get organised for the next day. If I was watching TV I was always folding washing or doing something. I'm used to being busy all the time and am addicted to activity.

When the babies were nine months old I went back to work. This helped me retain my sanity. I was recognised as a professional – not the triplet mum. I nursed nights and would sleep when they were at school. I was tired all the time.

The two people who helped me most were our GP and our pharmacist. The GP would make house calls all the time, for immunisations or sickness. I didn't want to abuse it but he'd get cross if I went into the clinic. The pharmacy would home deliver and pick up the script the GP had left at our place.

I have sacrificed my own needs but made informed choices. I wanted to give my children the best childhood possible. I would goal set endlessly. They're now reaching the end of Year 12. They all have goals that mean leaving home. I imagine I will be floundering. You bring up your children to be independent, accepted by society, understand boundaries and move on. Then it will all happen at once.

All the kids are close and I am proud that they are a bonded group. We had to work at it. If any of them felt 'lost' it was my second child who was three when the triplets were born. I used to say to her, 'There is something special in this life for you.'

I would take any anger out on my husband, not on my children. 'If you earned enough I wouldn't have to work so much, I wouldn't be so tired' – we needed a new car, house extensions, their constant illnesses and medication were all expenses. The government only gives you some financial support until they're at school – so you go to work to maintain some sort of standard. I also chose to send the five children to private schools.

The older girls got sick of being known as the triplets' sisters. Every Saturday morning was reserved for my time just with them. We'd either go shopping or to the movies. This was precious time and an investment in them and the whole family.

Being a triplet is a huge factor in shaping their personalities and their lives. They have a very close relationship. The bond and their ability to discuss and share intimacies is unmatched. They are a lot more mature than their older siblings at their age. They have the capacity to discuss, negotiate and compromise. I find them 'older' at seventeen than my other two.

They can debrief with each other – they're well respected by their peers. I've had no adolescent 'behaviour' issues at all. Having three 15-year-old children at the same time did present a number of challenges though. The middle years at high school were an intense time. The identity crises and lack of confidence that comes with adolescence is intensified when you've got three doing it. I had to be very careful to make time to sit with them as individuals, not as a group. I would take time in a quiet area to sit and talk one-on-one. Dealing with their personal issues, accompanied by their different personalities, takes more time for the parents.

Multiples have that constant point of comparison, particularly with body changes and one girl reaching puberty faster. My daughter felt there was something wrong with her because she didn't have boobs yet and other children at school would say, 'Your sister's got boobs, why haven't you?' Being a multiple in the eyes of other children you are recognised as different and they would be teased as a group. My argument was that they only share a birthday, you are you. Sometimes it was very heart wrenching when one of them felt different. The girls were advancing physically faster than my son. We tried to make light fun out of him not having whiskers yet. We used humour to let him know that we understood that he was struggling. The three of them really did support each other a lot during that time.

I feel a great sense of achievement and now I'm looking at what I want and where I want to be in five years. I'm not just thinking about what they need tomorrow.

My husband and I are strangers. We've tag-teamed—it's not been a combined 'together' effort. When he gets home, I'm off to work. Ongoing illnesses and never-ending bills doesn't make for a sex life. I feel like a single person and he feels the same.

I'm not sure about the quality of the marriage or if it's just a habit. I wonder what will happen when the children leave home. I sense we may go our own ways, but that's OK. We're both exhausted, and have no more to give each other. We both want something that neither of us can give.

TIPS FOR TRIPLET PARENTS

- Join AMBA.
- Email hom_families@yahoogroups.com.au – to add your family to the list of families with triplets and higher order multiples.
- Contact baby care companies for freebies.
- Ask friends and family to buy a gift for older children when the babies are born.
- Have a useful present list including subscriptions to healthy frozen meals, providing a cleaner or home-help, an extra fridge and encourage people to give disposable nappies
- Find a GP who will do home visits and bulk bill.
- Find a pharmacist who will deliver.
- Think about outsourcing work rather than having people do it in your home. This can include volunteers taking baskets of washing home and returning it clean.
- Organise help and draw up a roster – include someone who will make a commitment to overnight shifts.
- Advertise in your local paper, through local church or service club newsletters for potential volunteers.
- Australian Breastfeeding Association's booklet Breastfeeding Higher Order Multiples contains information from mothers who've breastfed their triplets.

Notes

The publishing details of some books mentioned below are given in full in Recommended Reading, page 339. General information came from discussions with parents and expectant parents of twins, health professionals and Professor David Hay and Dr Mark Umstad.

FINDING OUT

Statistics for difficulty conceiving are from ACCESS Australia's National Infertility Network. Further statistical information is from 'Monash IVF Infertility Update' brochures and from the 'Trends in Twinning, Triplet and other Multiple Births in Developed Countries 1972–1999' paper by Yoko Imaizumi presented at the 10th International Conference on Twin Studies, July 2001.

IVF eggs splitting information is from 'Monozygotic twinning rate after ovulation induction' paper by Catherine A. Derom, Robert M. Derom and Robert F. Vlietinck presented at the 10th International Conference on Twin Studies, July 2001.

Other information is from 'More Australian Births with Assisted Conception', myDr 2001.

Information about folate supplements increasing chances of conceiving twins is from 'Twin consequences face women who take folates', by Judith Whelan, *Sydney Morning Herald*, 14 March 2000.

Twins statistics from Australian Bureau of Statistics 'Confinements resulting in multiple births' 2000. Further facts and myths about twins were sourced from *Twins* by Lawrence Wright. Other facts and information were from Twins Magazine online www.twinsmagazine.com and the *Guinness Book of Records*.

Information for 'Twins are good for your health' was provided by the Australian Twin Registry.

PREGNANCY

'Week one to nine months' table is adapted from information on multiple foetal development in *The Multiple Pregnancy Sourcebook* by Nancy Bowers.

Twins headsize in uterus is taken from *When You're Expecting Twins, Triplets or Quads* by Dr Barbara Luke and Tamara Eberlein.

'Eating – what to eat and how much' has been adapted from 'Good Nutrition for Pregnancy – Twins and Triplets' booklet by Department of Nutrition and Dietetics, The Royal Women's Hospital, Melbourne. Other information came from *Guide to Nutrition During Pregnancy and Beyond*, The Vegetarian Society, UK, 1992.

Additional information on diet, bodyshape and size during a twin pregnancy is adapted from *When You're Expecting Twins, Triplets or Quads*, Chapter 3 'The Food Factor: eating right' and from *The Multiple Pregnancy Sourcebook*, Chapter 4 'Multiple Pregnancy, Nutrition: eating for everyone'.

Information on tests and procedures came from discussions with doctors and midwives, personal experiences, *Up The Duff* by Kaz Cooke, *The Multiple Pregnancy Sourcebook* by Nancy Bowers, 'Prenatal Diagnosis and Testing in Multiple Pregnancy', *When You're Expecting Twins, Triplets or Quads* by

Elizabeth M Bryan, 'Prenatal tests for moms-to-be of multiples' pp 141–147 and *What to Expect When You're Expecting* by Arlene Eisenberg, Heidi E. Murkoff and Sandee E. Hathaway, Harper Collins, 2000.

Information on resting, exercise and relaxation from *The Multiple Pregnancy Sourcebook*, Chapter 6 'Adapting your lifestyle with a multiple pregnancy'.

Eating discomforts and coping with difficulties information came from twin mothers, expectant twin mothers, *Up the Duff* and *What to Expect When You're Expecting*.

Possible complications came from Multiple Pregnancy Sourcebook, *When You're Expecting Twins, Triplet or Quads*, *Up the Duff*, and *What to Expect When You're Expecting*.

Additional information on chronic itching came from 'Obstetric Cholestasis', *The Obstetrician and Gynaecologist* (Journal) July 2000, Vol 2, No 3.

Small-for-dates babies information from 'Discordancy and Catch up Growth in Twins' paper by Mary L. Hediger, Dr Barbara Luke, Rita Misunas and Elaine Andersen presented at the 10th International Conference on Twin Studies, July 2001.

GETTING ORGANISED

Australian and New Zealand Standards information is from 'Keeping Baby Safe: a guide to nursery furniture' from the Ministerial Council on Consumer Affairs, Commonwealth of Australia, 1998.

Information on baby walkers is from 'Children and how they get harmed' by Greg Roberts, *The Age*, 18 July 2001, an article examining a report from the Injury Surveillance Unit, Mater Hospital, Brisbane. Information on private homes being the most dangerous came from the Child Accident Prevention Foundation of Australia.

Nappy analysis and the effect on the environment came from *Choice Magazine*, Australian Consumer Association, August 1999.

Car seat information came from 'Choosing and Using Restraints' booklet, Vic Roads 2000.

BIRTH

Optimum time for birth 35–38 weeks came from *When You're Expecting Twins, Triplets or Quads*. Induced labour, vaginal and caesarean and pain relief information came from personal experiences of twin mothers, theatre nurses, midwives, and *When You're Expecting Twins, Triplets or Quads*, and *The Multiple Pregnancy Sourcebook*.

HOSPITAL

Information is from interviews with midwives, physiotherapists and the experiences and mistakes from those who've done it.

'Essential Exercises for Good Health after Childbirth' leaflet by the Physiotherapy Department at The Queen Elizabeth Hospital, Woodville, South Australia

BREASTFEEDING

Information was taken from La Leche League newsletters and the Australian

Breastfeeding Association booklets, 'An introduction to breastfeeding', 'Breast and nipple care', 'Increasing your supply', 'Breastfeeding twins', 'Breastfeeding and hospitalisation', 'Gastro-oesophageal reflux and the breastfed baby', 'Breastfeeding after a caesarean birth', 'Expressing and storing breastmilk' and 'Breastfeeding women and work'.

Further information came from:
'Establishment of Twin Breastfeeding', Rosalie Donnelly RM, RN, EchN, The Australian Multiple Birth Association, 1995
'How to Succeed in Nursing Multiples With Really Trying' by Sharon Withers, Twins Magazine online, March/April 2000
'The Feeding Book', Child and Youth Health, Adelaide, 1999
'Breastfeeding – help!' *Medicine Today* Journal April 2001
La Leche League website www.lalecheleague.org
'Breast or bottle: what will you choose?' a pamphlet put together and distributed by the Australian Lactation Consultants Association, BFHI (Baby Friendly Hospitals) Australia, Australian College of Midwives and the Australian Breastfeeding Association
'Breastfeeding' and 'Breastfeeding Facts for Fathers', Child Health Fact Sheets by Department of Human Services 1997
When You're Expecting Twins, Triplets or Quads

BOTTLEFEEDING
Information was taken from: 'Breast or bottle: what will you choose?' pamphlet put together and distributed by the Australian Lactation Consultants Association, BFHI (Baby Friendly Hospitals) Australia, Australian College of Midwives and the Australian Breastfeeding Association, and 'Bottlefeeding Multiple Birth Babies', Catherine Worsnop, The Australian Multiple Birth Association, 1995.

HOME
Information was taken from conversations with psychologists and the following publications:
Australian Breastfeeding Association booklets, 'Survival plan' and 'Looking after yourself' and 'Gastro-oesophageal reflux and the breastfed baby'
'Settling your baby', Child and Youth Health, 1994
Baby Love
What to Expect in the First Year
'Crying', Parent Tip Sheet, Department of Human Services, 1997

MOTHERHOOD
Information from PANDA, psychologists and the following publications:
Australian Breastfeeding Association booklets, 'Survival plan' and 'Looking after yourself'
Mask of Motherhood and *Motherhood: making it work for you* by Jo Lamble and Sue Morris, Finch Publishing, Australia, 1999
'Missing Voices: what women say and do about depression after childbirth', R Small, S Brown, J Lumley and J Astbury, *Journal of Infant and Reproductive*

Psychology, 1994, Vol 12 p 89–103
National Institute of Mental Health Depression Awareness, Recognition and
  Treatment program at www.nimh.nih.gov

RELATIONSHIPS
Information was taken from psychologists and the following publications:
Wifework
The Mask of Motherhood
Twin and Triplet Psychology: A Professional Guide to Working with Multiples,
  edited by Audrey C Sandbank, Routledge, London & New York 1999.
When Partners Become Parents by Carolyn Pape Cowan and Phillip Cowan,
  Basic Books, New York, 1992, cited in Wifework

Strengthening your relationship steps were adapted from information from the
Department of Human Services.

SLEEP
Information on sleep came from Tweddle Child and Family Health Centre, SIDS
Australia and 'Sleep Right, Sleep Tight', 'Settling Your Baby' and Baby Love.

PRE-TERM BABIES
Information came from Australian Breastfeeding Association and their booklets,
'Expressing and storing breastmilk' and 'Breastfeeding your premature baby'.

Other publications consulted were:
'Hospitalisation: special care nursery and separate discharge', Joy Heads and
  Michelle Bonner, The Australian Multiple Birth Association 1995
'Early Arrivals', Monash Magazine Spring/Summer 2001. Victorian Infant
  Collaborative Study by Monash Medicine, Nursing and Health Science in
  conjunction with several Melbourne teaching hospitals
The Multiple Pregnancy Source Book
When You're Expecting Twins, Triplet and More

LOSING A TWIN
Information came from conversations with psychologists, SANDS and the
following publications:
Coping with Grief, McKissock, Hill of Content Press
The Multiple Pregnancy Sourcebook
Michael Carr-Gregg, Psychologist, Opinion, The Age, 14 January 2002

THE TWIN SITUATION
Twins
Twin and Triplet Psychology
'Solving the Birthday Party Dilemma', Australian Multiples Magazine, no 85
Dr Pat Preedy and Professor David Hay's website: www.twinsandmultiples.org
'Debate divided over whether to separate twins at school' article by Erica
  Cervini, The Sunday Age, 9 September 2001

Glossary

AMBA: Australian Multiple Birth Association

Amniocentesis: Test conducted between 15 and 20 weeks of pregnancy. It involves inserting a needle through the abdomen and drawing fluid which is then tested for potential chromosomal abnormalities.

Amniotic fluid: The fluid in the uterus surrounding unborn babies.

Australian and New Zealand Standards: The government regulatory safety standards for equipment used for babies and children.

Bloody show: A blood tinged mucous plug is released from the cervix when it begins to dilate. This mucous is called a 'bloody show'.

Breech presentation: The unborn baby's feet or buttocks lying closest to the cervix. This may mean the babies are born via caesarean section rather than a vaginal delivery.

Cervix: The narrow lower end of the uterus that opens into the vagina.

Chloasma: The dark pigmentation of the skin during pregnancy. It's often called the mask of pregnancy as it is usually visible around the face.

Colostrum: A yellow coloured liquid produced in the mother's breasts before breastmilk 'comes in'. It is highly nutritious and beneficial to newborns.

Carpal Tunnel Syndrome: A pinched nerve in the hand which can be caused by pregnancy associated weight gain.

Crying: Something parents of newborn twins find they do more often.

CVS – Chorionic Villus Sampling: A test for potential genetic disorders, conducted at 10 to 12 weeks gestation.

Diamniotic: A twin pregnancy with two separate amniotic sacs, each contains a baby.

Dichrionic: Two separate outer membranes, each surrounding one baby.

Dizygotic (DZ): Fraternal twins formed from two separate fertilised eggs.

Embryo: A baby developing in-utero after eight weeks since conception.

Engorgement: The breast swelling and tightness when a mothers milk 'comes in'.

Epidural: An injection of anaesthetic into the 'epidural' space of the spinal cord to numb the bodies nerves below the waist.

Episiotomy: An incision of the perineum (between the vagina and the anus) to enlarge the vaginal opening for birth and to prevent tearing. The incision is stitched following the birth.

Fraternal twins: Also known as dizygotic (DZ) twins. Two babies developed from two fertilised eggs in one pregnancy.

Foetal distress: Change in the foetal heartbeat or activity, including meconium stained amniotic fluid, signalling that a foetus is in possible danger.

Foetus: The term used to describe an unborn baby between formation of the embryo and the birth.

Frustration: An emotion usually felt more frequently by parents of twins.

Full term: Baby or babies born between 38 and 42 weeks gestation.

Gestation: The unborn baby's age counted in weeks, calculated from the first day of the mothers last menstrual period.

HCG – Human Chorionic Gonadotropin: A hormone produced by the chorion during pregnancy that is present in the mother's urine and blood.

HIV: Human Immuno Virus – the virus responsible for Acquired Immuno Deficiency Syndrome (AIDS).

Hypoglycaemia: Abnormally low blood sugar levels.

Identical twins: Twins that developed from one egg fertilised by one sperm, also known as MZ or monozygotic.

In utero: Occurring in the uterus before birth.

Induced labour: Labour brought on using a synthetic version of the hormone (oxytocin) that starts contractions.

IUGR – Intra Uterine Growth Restriction: Inadequate growth of a foetus compared to its gestational age (small-for-dates).

IVF – In Vitro Fertilisation: A fertility treatment in which eggs and sperm are fertilised in a laboratory and later transferred to a woman's uterus.

Isolette: A clear plastic box used as a bed for premature babies.

IV – Intravenous lines: A small needle or tube inserted into a vein to allow fluids into the blood stream.

Jaundice: The yellow appearance of a newborn's skin and eyes caused by a build up of bile pigment (bilirubin) in the blood.

Jelly belly: The remaining stomach skin after the babies are born, resulting from all that stretching. Also known as twin skin.

Kangaroo care: Skin to skin contact between the parent and babies.

Lactation consultant: A professional trained to give breastfeeding advice. Also known as a breastfeeding consultant.

Let-down reflex: The milk flows into ducts and collects in the area behind the nipples. Breastfeeding mothers may feel a tingling sensation.

Mastitis: A painful infection of the breast.

Meconium: The greenish, black, sticky substance passed as babies first bowel movements.

Monoamniotic: Two or more foetuses sharing one amniotic sac.

Monochorionic: Multiple foetuses sharing one outer membrane.

MZ – Monozygotic: See identical twins.

NICU – **Neonatal Intensive Care Unit:** The special nursery staffed and equipped to look after premature or sick newborn babies.

Nuchal screening test: A measuring of the thickness of the back of the foetal neck during ultrasound indicating likelihood of chromosomal abnormalities.

NZMBA: New Zealand Multiple Birth Association

Oligohydramniosis: Low levels of amniotic fluid in the amniotic sac.

Oxygen hood: A plastic hood used in NICU to supply oxygen to babies.

Oxytocin: The pituitary hormone causing uterine contractions and stimulating milk production.

PCA: Patient controlled analgesia.

Perineum: The area between the anus and the opening of the vagina.

Pitocin: The brand name for the synthetic hormone that induces labour.

Pelvic floor muscle exercises: The contracting and holding of the perineal muscles to strengthen the pelvic floor.

Placenta: The outer layer of the fertilised egg becomes the placenta. Its function is to exchange blood, oxygen and nutrients between the mother and the foetus.

Placental abruption: The placenta begins to separate from the uterus before the babies are born.

Placenta previa: The placenta lies low in the uterine wall, covering all or part of the cervix.

PND – Post Natal Depression: Strong feelings of sadness, anxiety or despair after childbirth. They can impair the mother's ability to function.

PNS – Parenteral Nutrition Supplement: A special formula given intravenously to very sick or premature babies. PNS contains essential nutrients for premature infants.

Polyhydramniosis: An excessive amount of amniotic fluid around the foetus.

Pre-eclampsia: Pregnancy induced hypertension where the mother may have rapid weight gain, swelling, a rise in blood pressure and protein in the urine.

Pre-term labour: Labour beginning prior to 37 weeks of pregnancy.

RDS – Respiratory Distress Syndrome: The collapse of lung tissue in premature babies with lungs that haven't yet developed enough surfactant.

RH factor: A protein in the red blood cells can lead to complications if it's in the blood of unborn babies.

Rupture of membranes: When the membrane surrounding the foetus breaks, often indicating the onset of labour. Also known as waters breaking.

SIDS – Sudden Infant Death Syndrome: The death of a healthy baby for unknown reasons.

Singleton: A single baby from a pregnancy.

Small-for-dates: Where the weight of a newborn is below the 10th percentile for gestational age.

Transverse presentation: A baby is lying sideways in the uterus.

Trimester: Pregnancy can be discussed in terms of the first, second and third trimester, each of around three months duration.

Twin skin: The soft jelly belly that can stay with the mother of twins for years after the birth.

Ultrasound: A test to view the internal organs of babies in the uterus. It uses high frequency sound waves that echo off the body and create a picture.

Umbilical cord: The connection between the foetus(es) and the placenta.

Vacuum/ventouse assisted birth: A suction cap is placed on the head of the unborn baby to help move the baby down the birth canal.

VBAC: Vaginal birth after a caesarean in a previous pregnancy.

Vanishing twin syndrome: The death and disappearance of a multiple during the first three months of pregnancy.

Vertex presentation: The baby is lying head down in the uterus.

Weaning: The decreasing or discontinuation of breastfeeding.

Zygote: A fertilised egg up to eight weeks following conception.

Recommended reading

Getting Pregnant by Robert Jansen, Allen & Unwin, Sydney, 1998

Up the Duff: The real guide to pregnancy by Kaz Cooke, Viking, Australia, 1999

Baby Love by Robyn Barker, Pan Macmillan, Australia, 2001

Twins,Triplets and More: Their nature, development and care by Elizabeth Bryan, Penguin, 1992

The Mighty Toddler by Robyn Barker, Pan Macmillan, Australia, 2001

Australian Baby and Toddler Meals by Robin Barker, Pan Macmillan, Australia, 1998

'*Sleep Right Sleep Tight*', Tweddle Child and Family Health Services

'*Settling your baby*', Child and Youth Health, 1994

Twin and Triplet Psychology: A professional Guide to Working With Multiples edited by Audrey C Sandbank, Routledge, London & New York, 1999

Twins by Lawrence Wright, Weidenfeld and Nicholson, London 1997

The Multiple Pregnancy Sourcebook: Pregnancy and first days with twins, triplets and more by Nancy Bowers, Contemporary Books, 2001

The Mask of Motherhood: How motherhood changes everything and why we pretend it doesn't by Susan Maushart, Vintage, Sydney, 1998

Wifework: What marriage really means by Susan Maushart, Penguin, 2001

Parenting by Heart by Pinky McKay, Lothian, 2000

Kidwrangling by Kaz Cooke, Viking, Australia, 2000

Resources

FINDING OUT IT'S TWINS
Australian Multiple Birth Association (AMBA)
PO Box 105
COOGEE NSW 2023

State contacts:
NSW 02 9875 2404
SA 08 8364 0433
VIC 03 9513 2050
www.amba.org.au
secretary@amba.org.au

New Zealand Multiple Birth Association (NZMBA)
(50 Local branches)
PO Box 1258
Wellington
New Zealand
www.nzmba.info
0800 4 TWINS ETC / 0800 489 467 (within NZ only)

Parents without Partners
NSW 02 9853 3269
VIC 03 9836 3211
www.pwp.freeyellow.com

IVF Parents Support Group:
ACCESS IVFP Options
PO Box 959
Parramatta NSW 2124
Australia
info@access.org.au
02 9670 2380

Australian Twin Registry
Level 2, 723 Swanston Street
Carlton VIC 3053
Australia
Freecall 1800 037 021
dph-twins@unimelb.edu.au
www.twins.org.au

Health Insurance Commission
www.hic.gov.au
02 6124 6333

Sources of twin type testing (zygosity testing):
Scientist, Molecular Biology
Victorian Institute of Forensic Medicine
Dept of Forensic Medicine, Monash University
57-83 Kavanagh St
Southbank VIC 3006
03 9684 4337
dna@vifp.monash.edu.au
www.vifp.monash.edu.au

Genetic Technologies Corporation Pty Ltd
PO Box 115
Fitzroy VIC 3065
VIC 03 9415 7688
NSW 02 9906 3626
gtc@genetictechnologies.com.au
www.genetictechnologies.com.au

PREGNANCY
To find hospitals with Multiple Pregnancy Clinics, contact your nearest hospital.
Royal Women's Hospital, Multiple Pregnancy Clinic
132 Grattan St
Carlton VIC 3053
03 9344 2709

Mater Mothers' Hospital
Raymond Tce
South Brisbane QLD 4101
07 3840 8844
fchan@mater.org.au
Fun Yee Chan, Professor in Maternal Fetal Medicine

King Edward Memorial Hospital
374 Bagot Road
Subiaco WA 6008
08 9340 2222
jdickinson@obsgyn.uwa.edu.au
Jan Dickinson, Associate Professor, School of Women's and Infants' Health

Support for complicated pregnancies
www.sidelines.org

Support for complicated multiple pregnancies
www.monoamniotic.org

Back care
Australian Physiotherapy Association 03 9534 9400
www.physiotherapy.asn.au
Australian Society of Teachers of the Alexander Technique (AUSTAT) 1800
339 571
www.alexandertechnique.org.au
Chiropractors' Association of Australia 1800 075 003
www.chiropractors.asn.au

GETTING ORGANISED
Australian Family Assistance Office
13 6150
www.familyassist.gov.au

Kidsafe – the Child Accident Prevention Foundation of Australia
VIC 03 9345 6471
NSW 02 9845 0890
www.kidsafe.org.au

'Keeping baby safe – a guide to nursery furniture' booklet:
Consumer Affairs
www.consumer.gov.au

Poisons Information Centre
13 1126

Online grocery shopping:
  www.colesonline.com.au
  www.woolworths.com.au
  www.greengrocer.com.au
  www.shopfast.com.au

Puddle feeders, baby slings, literature:
www.breastfeeding.asn.au/products/mothersdirect.html

Pillows to help breastfeed twins, double slings and other products from US:
www.doubleblessings.com
www4.tpg.com.au/dicer/

BREASTFEEDING
Australian Breastfeeding Association
1818–1822 Malvern Road
East Malvern VIC 3145
Australia
03 9885 0855
info@breastfeeding.asn.au
www.breastfeeding.asn.au

Breastfeeding helplines
ACT/Southern NSW   02 6258 8928
NSW   02 9639 8686
QLD   07 3844 8977/8166
SA/NT   08 8411 0050
TAS (Nth)   03 6331 2799
TAS (Sth)   03 6223 2609
VIC   03 9885 0653
WA   08 9340 1200

La Leche League New Zealand
04 471 0690
24 hour counselling service
www.lalecheleague.org/LLLNZ

EZ-2-Nurse Twins Nursing & Bottle Feeding Pillow
Small Blessings www4.tpg.com.au/dicer/
02 8824 3313

HOME
Lifeline 13 1114
Parent Help Lines (24 hours)
QLD   1300 301 300
VIC   13 2289
SA   1300 364 100

Karitane
NSW:Telephone advice 24 hours
FREECALL (country areas) 1800 677 961
Sydney metro 02 9794 1852
www.swsahs.nsw.gov.au/karitane/

Tresillian (Royal Society for the Welfare of Mothers & Babies)
NSW: Parent Helpline 24 hours
        (country areas) 1800 637 357
        Sydney metro 02 9787 5255

Child Care Access Hotline
1800 670 305
Royal NZ Plunket Society (maternal and child health nurses)
04 471 0177
www.plunket.org.nz

SLEEP
'Settling your baby' booklet:
Child and Youth Health
295 South Terrace

Adelaide SA 5000
08 8303 1551
www.cyh.com

SLEEP SCHOOLS
Tweddle Child and Family Health Service
53 Adelaide St
Footscray VIC 3011
03 9689 1577

Tresillian Family Care Centres
02 9787 0800

Karitane Residential
02 9794 1800

MOTHERHOOD
PANDA
270 Church St
Richmond 3121
03 9428 4600
panda@vicnet.net.au
www.panda.org.au
This is a self-help support association for women who experience postnatal or antenatal depression and their families.

Program for mothers managing guilt, anxiety, depression or anger:
www.beingamother.com
03 9882 7958

www.beyondblue.org.au
National depression initiative
Information for Australian mothers:
www.motherinc.com.au
www.mumstheword.com.au

Quality Childcare
1300 136 554
www.ncac.gov.au/

RELATIONSHIPS
Relationships Australia
1300 364 277
www.relationships.com.au (including online counselling service)
Pride and Joy: a resource for prospective lesbian parents in Victoria, produced by the Royal Women's Hospital
www.rwh.org.au/wellwomens/whic.cfm?doc_id=4623

PRE-TERM BABIES
Premie Press
PO Box 547
KEW VIC 3101
03 9817 7552
A quarterly magazine for the parents of pre-term babies. To contact the
publisher, email carol.newnham@austin.org.au.

Parents of Premature Babies
www.preemie-l.org

LOSING A TWIN
SANDS Australia
National contact 03 9899 0217
www.sands.org.au
*Support and understanding following the death of a baby from the time of
conception through to infancy – contacts are available in each Australian state.*

Bonnie Babes Foundation
03 9758 2800
enquiry@bbf.org.au
www.bbf.org.au/
*24 hour grief counselling for families who have lost a baby during pregnancy or
shortly after birth*

Australian Multiple Birth Association (AMBA) – Bereavement Support Group
PO Box 105
COOGEE NSW 2023
www.amba.org.au   bereavement@amba.org.au

State contacts:
NSW 02 9875 2404
VIC 03 9513 2050

SIDs and KIDS
1300 308 307
Or write to GPO Box 9914 in your capital city
www.sidsandkids.org

Pen–Parents of Australia
PO Box 574
Belconnen ACT 2616
penparents@sidsandkids.org

Twin and Multiple Loss Support
PO Box 51–984
Pakuranga, Auckland NZ

Center for Loss in Multiple Birth (CLIMB) Inc
www.climb-support.org/
For parents of multiples dealing with loss, prematurity and special needs
www.synspectrum.com/multiplicity.html

For parents of twins who have lost their co-twin at birth or shortly after
www.upnaway.com/~junem

Australian Twin to Twin Transfusion Syndrome Support Group
PO Box 1343
Carindale QLD 4152
www.twin-twin.org/aust_contacts.htm

Australian Twinless – contact group for any twin who has lost their twin by
whatever means, and the parents/carers of such twins
http://groups.yahoo.com/group/AustralianTwinless/

Twinless Twins Support Group International
www.twinlesstwins.org

For parents of multiples who have experienced the death of a twin or some of
their multiple birth babies/children
www.erichad.com

THE TWIN SITUATION
Speech Pathology Australia ph 03 9642 4899
www.speechpathologyaustralia.org.au/

For further information on twin identity, schooling and language development
checklist:
www.twinsandmultiples.org

For information about parenting of multiples:
www.multiples.about.com/library/weekly/

International Society for Twin Studies (includes link to the Declaration of
Rights and Statement of Needs for Twins and Higher Order Multiples)
www.ists.qimr.edu.au/

National Organization of Mothers of Twins Club (USA)
www.nomotc.org
Twin Stuff – web community for twins, triplets and their families
www.twinstuff.com/

TAMBA (Twins & Multiple Birth Association UK)
www.tamba.org.uk/

TWINS Magazine Online
www.twinsmagazine.com

Twin Days – Twinsburg Ohio
www.twinsdays.org

Yahoo! Twins listings:
dir.yahoo.com/Society_and_Culture/Families/Multiple_Births/Twins/

For online catalogue of twin products:
www.morethan1.com

For products and information for multiple birth families:
www.twinshelp.com

The Center for the Study of Multiple Birth
www.multiplebirth.com

Twins: A Parent's Guide
www.vh.org/Patients/IHB/Peds/General/Twins/Twins.html

Triplet Resources

AMBA Triplets and more (Higher Order Multiples support)
hom@amba.org.au
www.amba.org.au

Email address for other parents of triplets and higher order multiples
hom_families@yahoogroups.com.au

Acknowledgements

FOR THEIR PROFESSIONAL EXPERTISE

Dr Mark Umstad, Head Obstetrician, Multiple Pregnancy Clinic, The Royal Women's Hospital in Melbourne

Robin Barker, Maternal health guru, for inspiration and heaps of help

Professor David Hay, School of Psychology, Curtin University and Patron AMBA

Dr John Hopper and Maggie Lenaghan at the Australian Twin Registry

Dr Louise Van Geyzel

Dr Charmaine Gittleson

Finbar Hopkins RN

Kerryn Roem, Dietitian, The Royal Women's Hospital in Melbourne

Jane Davies, Kirsty Greenwood and Kate Mortenson at the Australian Breastfeeding Association

Betty Chetcuti, psychologist

Gina Ralston, Education Network Coordinator at Tweddle Family Services

Deborah Herz, women's health physiotherapist

Sue Breheny at Monash IVF

Cathy Vellacott, CEO, Australian Multiple Birth Association (AMBA)

Helen Coburn, South Eastern Multiple Birth Association (SEMBA)

Gladys Billing and Gillian Dibley, New Zealand Multiple Birth Association (NZMBA)

Nerrida Mulvey and Dorothy Ford at SIDS Australia

Liz Senior and Terrie Hollingsworth at PANDA

Pinky McKay, parenting advisor

Dr Elizabeth Bryan

SPECIAL PEOPLE

Sue Hines and Andrea McNamara for publishing a humble but worthy book.

Jenny Lord (editor), Andrew Cunningham (designer) and Pauline Haas (typesetter) for making it all into a book.

Leith Condon, Melinda Dundas and Jacqui Gray for listening, for their enthusiasm, constructive advice and encouragement.

Rebecca Perovic for her quiet assistance.

Shirley Accheni, Liz Allen, Wendy Bailey, Kellie Ciccocioppo, Jacinta Covington, Robin Culph, Melinda Eales, Helen Eggleton, Trina Eldering, Cecile Ferguson, Louise Green, Kerri Griffin, Daniela Hongel, Paula Hurley, Linda Johnson, Donna Lehmann, Lynn Lelean, Rebecca Lloyd, Jane Longmire, Donna McKay, Bert Newton, Helen Owens, Libby Paholski, Adrianne Perry, Eliot Perry, Erica Ryan, Jacqui Saultry, Sandy Shew, Sarah Smith, Cindy Trewin, Michael Vardon, Ros Williamson and Merridy Wilson, Richard, Matilda, Edward and Kyra Wilson.

VERY SPECIAL PEOPLE WHO WORKED HARD FOR US WHEN THEY HAD NEITHER THE TIME NOR THE ENERGY
Louise Ajani for her sharp mind and honesty.
Hilary Bonney for reading and re-reading.
Andrea Wilson for her strength, wisdom and poignant advice.

FOR GIVING US A TWIN AND TRIPLET PERSPECTIVE
Kylie Miller and Kadi Morrison

FOR HAVING TWINS, LETTING US INTO THEIR FAMILIES AND CONTRIBUTING THEIR EXPERIENCES
Katie Biggin and Bruce, Mali, Luka & Fergus
Jane Buckley and Michael Dann, Darcy, Jesse & Alexis
Tania Callaghan and Jim, Will & Sam
Carol Constantine and Colin, Alex, Tony & Ben
Jane Garrow and Jonathon Muller, Evie & Rosie
Ray Gibson, Audrey & Hannah
Charmaine Gittleson and Grant, Jules & Wade
Cheryl Hall and Andrew Kaleski, Ellen, Sophia & Grace
Sharon and Grant Higgins, Jack, Morgan & Kelsey
Finbar Hopkins and Loy Lichtman, Niamh & Aoife
Kearin and Rob Lee, Jayden, Jarryn, Reidan, Shiarne & Tanashae
Paul Maruff, Stella, Ari & Louis
Colleen and Dallas McCosh, Oliver, Isabel & Ashleigh
Michelle Moore and Mark Miller, Tom & Gus
Toni O'Sullivan and Tony, Lachlan & Harry
Belinda Ricardo and Craig, Kayla, Georgia & Zoe
Michele Riggs and Murray, Tiffany, Elisha, Charlotte, Phoebe & Zachary
Rebekah Robertson and Greg Stone, George & Harry
Susanne and Manfred Stoeghofer, Jesse, Perry, Mark & Richard
Caroline Tehan and Chris James, Rory & Albert
Jayne Timms and Steve, Liam, Matthew, Riley, Kegan & Ruby
Kylie Beatson, Tammy Davie, Yolande Dickson-Smith, Carlene Dowie, Paula-Jane Fergusson, Verna Fisher, Clare Gleeson-McGuire, Eugenia Gurrieri, Nicky Kyrou, Kay Libson, Toni Long, Suzie Martens, Janine McAuley, Kristy Morrison, Katie O'Callaghan, Nyomi Ord, Melinda Purtill, Victoria Ramirez, Stephanie Renton, Lucy Sporne, Kathy Stack, Debra Simpson, Tenille Telford, Sue-Ellen Timcke, Carmel Tonkin, Rosemary Vine, Sarah Wells and Catherine Wiles-Harrell.

Index

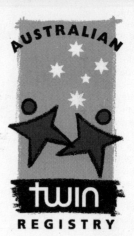